THE

ANSWER

TO

CANCER

. . . .

STOP IT BEFORE IT STARTS • ARREST IT IN
ITS EARLIEST STAGES • KEEP IT FROM COMING BACK

THE

ANSWER

TO

CANCER

• • • • • • • • •

Carolyn D. Runowicz, M.D., and Sheldon H. Cherry, M.D.
with Dianne Partie Lange

RODALE

© 2004 by Carolyn D. Runowicz, M.D., and Sheldon H. Cherry, M.D.

Printed in the United States of America
Rodale Inc. makes every effort to use acid-free (∞), recycled paper (♻).

Book design by Susan P. Eugster

Library of Congress Cataloging-in-Publication Data

Runowicz, Carolyn D.
    The answer to cancer / Carolyn D. Runowicz and Sheldon H. Cherry ; with
Dianne Partie Lange.
        p.   cm.
    Includes index.
    ISBN 1–57954–730–3 hardcover
    1. Cancer—Popular works.   2. Cancer—Chemoprevention—Popular works.
3. Cancer—Prevention—Popular works. I. Cherry, Sheldon H. II. Lange, Dianne.
III. Title.
RC263.R86   2004
616.99'405—dc22   2004010673

Distributed to the trade by Holtzbrinck Publishers

2   4   6   8   10   9   7   5   3   1   hardcover

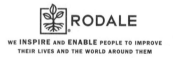

WE **INSPIRE** AND **ENABLE** PEOPLE TO IMPROVE
THEIR LIVES AND THE WORLD AROUND THEM

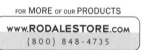

FOR MORE OF OUR PRODUCTS
WWW.RODALESTORE.COM
(800) 848-4735

To our patients and families

Contents

ACKNOWLEDGMENTS

For their individual contributions in shaping the vision and content of this book, our special thanks go to Dianne Partie Lange, Ellen Levine, Fern Williams, Tami Booth, and Susan Berg.

—SHELDON AND CAROLYN

THE

CANCER

PROBLEM

CANCER SCARES US, AND FOR GOOD REASON. It kills more people between ages 45 and 64 than anything else. Experts estimate that it soon will surpass heart disease as the number one cause of death in the United States.

It scares us, too, because it often comes without warning. Although cancer typically develops over many years, we may not discover it until it causes symptoms. By then, the window of opportunity for cure is closing fast.

Even when we detect cancer early on, it has the power to frighten us. Treatments can be harsh, and the threat of a recurrence hangs like a cloud of uncertainty over the future.

Finally, cancer scares us because the risk factors seem to be everywhere. Cancer-causing agents lurk in the air we breathe, in the food we eat—even within our own bodies, in the genes we inherit.

Maybe because it's so frightening, some of us prefer to put the possibility of cancer out of our minds, crossing our fingers that it never touches us or those we love. We'd be smart to change our strategy. Yes, cancer is a formidable foe, but it is not invulnerable. We can do more than simply hope to avoid it. We can take action to lower our risk.

A NEW FOCUS FOR RESEARCH

The more we learn about the process that sets the stage for cancer, the more we learn about methods that can alter its course. Since this process usually occurs over many years, we have many opportunities to disrupt it. Scientists are making great strides in determining how we can stop cancer before it gets a foothold in the body.

In medical terms, an action that switches off cancer formation or eliminates a precancer is known as an intervention. Some of the most exciting cancer research going on today is showing that interventions work. For instance, women who have undergone treatment for breast cancer can take a drug to block the hormonal signals that could stimulate a recurrence. For men, a drug commonly prescribed to relieve benign prostate enlargement also can lower prostate cancer risk. And a topical cream that clears up actinic keratoses—brown spots caused by the sun—helps prevent skin cancer as well. (For that matter, so does removing the spots surgically.)

Since the passage of the National Cancer Act in 1971, there has been a government-backed nationwide movement to control cancer. But the impetus to focus on prevention really got going in 1981, with the publication of a landmark study whose authors concluded that most cancers affecting Americans are avoidable. According to the authors, Sir Richard Doll and Sir Richard Peto, about one-third of cancers result from smoking, one-third from diet, and one-third from environmental and occupational causes.

A few years before Doll and Peto's famous paper, Michael B. Sporn, M.D., conducted a study on the use of vitamin A and its derivatives to slow the cancer process. His work with these particular substances, which he called retinoids, gave birth to a whole new concept: chemoprevention.

Nearly 2 decades later, scientific proof that drugs could prevent cancer in humans was mounting rapidly. In the late 1990s, researchers found that a vaccine against hepatitis B dramatically reduced the incidence of liver cancer in Asia, where the disease had been very prevalent. In 1998, a study of tamoxifen—already found to head off recurrences in breast cancer survivors—showed that the drug could reduce risk by 40 percent in women especially susceptible to the disease. Retinoids, the vitamin A derivatives that led Dr. Sporn to shape the concept of chemoprevention, proved effective in getting rid of oral precancers. And nonsteroidal anti-inflammatory drugs, or NSAIDs, were useful in keeping colon polyps—which can turn cancerous—from coming back.

To date, the FDA has approved a few drugs that help prevent cancer by treating precancers. Among them are BCG, for recurrent bladder tumors; topical fluorouracil, for actinic keratoses; tamoxifen, for women with ductal carcinoma in situ (abnormal cells that have not yet spread beyond the lining of the breast duct); and celecoxib, for colon polyps.

Finding other drugs that could prevent cancer has become a very active area of study. In 1998, the National Cancer Institute established the Chemoprevention Implementation Group to set research priorities. This group, in turn, created the Rapid Access to Preventive Intervention Development (RAPID) program, whose mission is to speed the process of bringing research from the laboratory to clinical trial, and to recommend other strategies for identifying and testing preventive agents.

SEPARATING FACT FROM FICTION

Just as there probably is no single drug or treatment that will cure cancer, there probably is no magic bullet that will prevent it, either. Each person has a unique genetic code, a unique lifestyle and environment, and a unique willingness to do what's necessary to maintain his or her health. For this reason, everyone must look at their own situation and make their own decisions about what's necessary to lower their cancer risk.

In this book, we hope to provide you with information to assess your own risk and make appropriate choices. We also hope to spare you the time, energy, and expense of trying things that have not proved helpful and that in fact may be harmful.

Sometimes it seems that every day brings a new headline about a nutrient, supplement, or drug that prevents cancer. A single study may add to the body of scientific evidence, but by itself, it is not proof. Several studies, including very large ones, are necessary to determine whether a particular intervention actually works.

Showing that certain foods and dietary habits are effective preventives can be especially challenging. Scientists struggle to maintain control over what their human subjects eat. And the people themselves don't always remember what they eat, either.

Because the cancer process takes so long, evaluating the impact of certain nutrients also can be difficult. Thus far, studies that meet key scientific criteria are not too encouraging. In fact, two such trials found that rather than help to prevent cancer, extra doses of key nutrients encourage cancer growth or fail to inhibit precancers. For example, in a study evaluating vitamin E and beta-carotene, supplements of both nutrients promoted rather than prevented lung cancer in male smokers.

This is our objective—to provide a reality check about what you can and can't do to lower your cancer risk. Along the way, we intend to clear up some common cancer prevention myths. Perhaps most pervasive at the moment is the notion that all kinds of supplements have preventive powers. Patients routinely come to us with bags full of pills or long lists of supplements that they hope will protect them from a cancer diagnosis. Right now, we have only preliminary evidence to suggest that these products might do what they claim. What we do know for certain, with regard to nutrition and cancer prevention, is this: First, eating fruits and vegetables reduces risk; and second, being overweight—which often stems from poor dietary habits—increases risk.

In writing this book, we have made every effort to distinguish between what is proven to help prevent cancer, what no longer holds promise, and what shows promise but is not yet proven. Much remains to be discovered, and many studies are pointing in exciting new directions. But if you're contemplating paying for certain tests, taking certain supplements or medications, or changing your diet or lifestyle, you should start with an accurate picture of the current "state of the science" in cancer prevention.

We want to stress again that assessing cancer risk is a very individualized task. You are a unique genetic package, and your risk factors are different from those of your neighbors, your friends, even your siblings. What's important to remember is that while some risk factors (like your age, ethnicity, and family history) are beyond your control, others (like eating a high-fat diet or not exercising) are yours to change. Throughout this book, you'll learn how to modify your risk profile and how to evaluate your risk for cancer in general, as well as for the nine most common forms of the disease.

THE KEY TO STAYING CANCER-FREE

The study of how to modify the cancer process has snowballed in recent years. Today certain professional conferences and medical journals focus exclusively on prevention. It's the new frontier of cancer research. Of course, developing new cancer treatments is an ongoing priority. But the most exciting and promising developments are in early detection and prevention.

For example, researchers have produced a vaccine to protect against infection with the virus that causes cervical cancer. They also have devised a method for catching early on the cellular changes that could lead to breast cancer. Various drugs excel in preventing breast, prostate, and colon cancers—and scores more are in the research pipeline.

Scientists the world over are scrutinizing different dietary components to determine why fruits, vegetables, soy products, and the polyphenols in green tea—among other foods and food-derived substances—are such potent cancer fighters. Perhaps they work best for people who are genetically programmed to respond to them. Maybe certain combinations are more beneficial than others. Or maybe they share a single, common substance that's responsible for their cancer-fighting potential. As the answers come to light, the face of cancer prevention will transform.

We're convinced that the solution to the cancer problem lies in detecting precancerous changes before they mushroom to full-blown cancer, and in stopping the cancer process from ever starting. With this two-pronged approach, you can do so much to dramatically lower your risk. And the more you learn about cancer prevention now, the better equipped you will be to take advantage of groundbreaking new measures that we suspect will be making headlines in the near future.

· · · · · · · ● · ·

PART I

A CANCER

PRIMER

· · · · · · • · ·

CHAPTER 1

WHAT

IS

CANCER?

. . . .

EVERY CELL IN THE BODY IS PROGRAMMED to perform a certain job, depending on which organ it is part of. With the exception of brain and nerve cells, the rest continually develop, divide, die, and are replaced with newly formed cells.

It's believed that cells replicate a finite number of times, though just what determines their life spans remains a mystery. In any event, if the genetic machinery that directs a cell's division to proceed on a predetermined schedule goes awry, the cell may continue growing, and at a faster rate than normal. Similarly, a cell that experiences a malfunction in its genetic program to self-destruct may keep dividing indefinitely, rather than dying.

Nobel prize–winning scientist H. Robert Horvitz, Ph.D., an expert in the genetic intricacies of normal cell death, succinctly describes cancer as a change in the equilibrium between cell division or growth and cell death. "If you have too much cell division, you get an increase in cell number; if you have too little cell death, you also get an increase in cell number," Dr. Horvitz explains. "Either can lead to cancer."

Cells divide too often or refuse to die because of a genetic error, and usually more than one. Fortunately, the body has the ability to protect itself against a cell that contains flawed genetic messages. For instance, natural killer cells—which are components of a healthy immune system—will detect and eliminate a mutated, misbehaving cell. But sometimes the body's search-and-destroy mechanisms fail, and a malformed cell continues to divide, generating more and more copies of itself.

Although these renegade cells differ slightly from one another, they tend to cluster together, forming a mass or tumor. On the whole, they're an aggressive bunch, bullying and pushing their way into healthy tissues. Eventually a tumor can become so large that the affected organ can't do its job. Or a tumor may press on neighboring structures, obstructing some vital function or causing pain.

What's more, tentacles of the cancer cells can extend from the tumor into adjacent tissues, as well as into blood and lymph vessels. Sometimes the cells break free and spread through these circulating channels to distant organs, where they form more clusters of abnormal cells and a secondary cancer. This spreading process is known as metastasis.

The further cancer progresses, the less likely it is to be stopped. Once it has spread, or metastasized, to other parts of the body, successful treatment becomes very difficult.

NOT ALL CANCERS ARE ALIKE

The progression from that first cluster of abnormal cells to a detectable tumor may take years. Cancer cells, being outsiders, follow no rules. They don't grow steadily and smoothly in a coordinate way, like healthy cells with flawless genetic messages. Instead, they tend to rest and grow, rest and grow.

But some cancers, when they are in a growth stage, can become quite large quite fast. They develop and spread so quickly that they may not be discovered until they are so large that they produce life-threatening symptoms.

Even a single form of cancer can manifest many different ways. For instance, one man may have prostate cancer all his life, but it grows so slowly that it doesn't produce symptoms and never spreads beyond his prostate gland, where it began. In fact, his cancer may remain undetected until he dies from some other cause. Another man may learn that he has advanced prostate cancer less than a year after a normal screening test. Ultimately, he may die from the disease.

Whether they grow quickly or slowly, not all tumors can be felt. If one is buried deep within the chest or abdomen, for instance, a person will have no clue that it's there unless it begins to interfere with some vital function or produces symptoms.

Fortunately, researchers have developed screening tests to find these hidden cancers before they reach advanced stages, as well as to detect abnormalities before they become full-fledged cancers. They're called screening tests because they're performed on healthy people who have no symptoms, for the sole purpose of looking for cancer or a condition that could lead to cancer. Screening tests that detect precancerous conditions are an essential part of cancer prevention. We will discuss tests that doctors now use, and those that researchers still are perfecting, throughout this book.

RECOGNIZING THE ENEMY

It has been said that cancer is more than 100 different diseases because it varies according to the type of cell that's involved and the organ that is home to those cells. Despite this inherent diversity, all cancers share four fundamental characteristics.

1. CANCER BEGINS WITH THE BODY'S OWN CELLS. The cause—that is, whatever alters the genetic message within a cell— may come from outside the body. But the tumor itself is a cluster of cells.

2. THE CELLS GROW OUT OF CONTROL AND DON'T DIE. If a cancer is not detected and removed—or if its growth is not stopped with chemotherapy or radiation therapy—the cells will continue to divide.

3. THE CELLS FROM THE TUMOR MAY EXTEND INTO SURROUNDING TISSUES AND ORGANS, OFTEN DESTROYING THEM IN THE PROCESS. Even if this occurs, a cancer may not be fatal. The key is to excise all or part of the affected tissue, removing any trace of cancer cells. As extra insurance, this surgery often is followed by chemotherapy or radiation therapy to kill any cells that may have escaped detection.

Later in the book, you'll learn how some drugs can help prevent a recurrence of cancer when taken after treatment for the disease. Doctors refer to this as chemoprevention. They use the same term to describe drugs that stop the development of cancer in the first place.

4. THE CELLS CAN TRAVEL FAR FROM THE ORIGINAL TUMOR. Eventually, cancer cells enter the circulatory and lymphatic systems. From there, they spread to other areas of the body and begin to grow at those distant sites.

Because some 200 different kinds of cells exist in the body, doctors identify cancers according to the cells from which they originate. Every cell falls into one of four general categories:

- Epithelial cells, which comprise skin and line the passageways of the breasts, lungs, stomach, intestine, bladder, ovaries, uterus, and prostate

- Connective tissue cells, such as those that form cartilage, bone, muscle, and blood vessels

- Blood-forming cells, which make up the bone marrow

- Nerve cells, which include those in the brain and the body

Let's suppose that a doctor diagnoses a patient with epithelial carcinoma. In layperson's language, this means a cancer that involves the epithelial cells. Doctors also may describe tumors according to the function of the cells. For instance, an adenocarcinoma arises from secreting glands, such as those that form in the breasts from epithelial tissue.

Tests are available to determine the aggressiveness of a particular cancer, as well as appropriate treatment options. Although these tests are important, they can be done only after a cancer has been discovered. Researchers are working to identify markers that alert doctors to the presence of a cancer or precancer that consists of just a few cells. Then, even if the cancer is aggressive, the cells can be removed or destroyed before a tumor develops.

A good example of this type of test is the Papanicolaou smear, or Pap test, which has been in use since the 1950s. This routine screening test for women detects abnormal cells on the cervix that are likely to become malignant. More recently, researchers have been working on tests to examine breast fluid for cancer cells, and stool samples for abnormal cells from the colon lining. The tests are under evaluation to determine their accuracy in discovering precancerous conditions and their practicality for widespread clinical use.

How Cancer Begins

As complicated as cancer is, and as confusing and complex as the names of the many different kinds of cancer are, the simple fact is that the disease begins with a single cell. From there, it follows a well-choreographed process consisting of three key steps: initiation, promotion, and progression. Each of these plays a crucial role in cancer prevention. In particular, measures such as risk control, early detection, and chemoprevention are likely to be most effective during the first two steps.

The following discussion gets a bit technical, so you may want to skip over it for now and come back to it when you're reading about a specific aspect of cancer prevention. It provides the necessary background for understanding why some things protect against cancer and, perhaps equally important, why other things don't. If you understand how the disease develops in the first place, you'll be better able to take action to lower your risk.

INITIATION

All cancers begin with a mistake within a cell's chromosomes, which serve as the containers of the cell's genetic material, or DNA (short for deoxyribonucleic acid). The mistake may appear in the chromosome itself, or it could turn up in a gene—a segment of DNA—within the chromosome.

DNA consists of a long chain of chemicals tightly wound within the chromosome. The strands of DNA in each of our 23 pairs of chromosomes contain between 30,000 and 40,000 genes.

While a mistake, or mutation, in a gene may be inherited from a parent, it's more likely to occur spontaneously in the course of cell division. Or it could be the result of some external factor. A physical injury

Chromosome with DNA

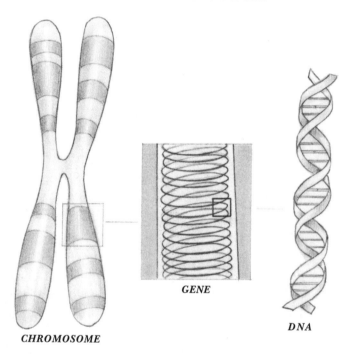

GENE

DNA

CHROMOSOME

DNA (DEOXYRIBONUCLEIC ACID) IS A THREAD OF FOUR PRECISELY ORDERED CHEMICALS COILED UP WITHIN EACH CHROMOSOME IN A CELL'S NUCLEUS. (EACH CELL CONTAINS 46 CHROMOSOMES.) THE FOUR CHEMICALS THAT MAKE UP DNA JOIN EACH OTHER, FORMING A TWISTING, LADDERLIKE STRUCTURE DESCRIBED AS A DOUBLE HELIX. UNITS OF DNA ALONG THIS LADDER, OR GENES, CONTAIN A CODE THAT INSTRUCTS THE CELL TO MAKE A SPECIFIC PROTEIN.

such as bombardment with radiation can cause a mutation. So can a viral infection or chronic inflammation. For example, in ulcerative colitis—inflammation of the intestinal tract—cells divide very rapidly, increasing the possibility for error. A mutation also can be linked to a chemical, like the ones in tobacco smoke.

Anything that's responsible for triggering a genetic mutation that eventually can turn into cancer is known as an initiator or a carcinogen. You'll learn more about carcinogens in part 2, when we discuss specific cancers.

The good news is, most of the mutations that affect DNA are corrected by the body's built-in repair mechanisms, which also are under genetic control. The injured DNA can be replaced with a healthy section, using what might best be described as a cellular patch kit. Enzymes that remove certain kinds of damage travel to the site of the mutation to make the necessary repairs.

Unfortunately, mutations also can occur in the genes that govern these repair mechanisms, as well as in the genes that control a cell's growth or death. In particular, mistakes in the genes responsible for cell growth, called oncogenes, can lay the groundwork for cancer. This is because as mutations accumulate, the opportunity for oncogenes to become hyperactive increases as well. A protein that's produced by oncogenes instructs cells to reproduce endlessly.

So far, scientists have identified more than 100 different oncogenes. Usually several take part in the cancer process. Sometimes they're switched on by external factors, such as substances in tobacco smoke and the ultraviolet radiation in sunlight.

Some oncogenes tend to be associated with certain cancers. One example is RAS, an oncogene that plays a role in colorectal cancer.

Mutations even appear in genes whose sole purpose is to stop tumors from forming and/or growing—hence the name tumor suppressor genes. One such gene that is especially well-known to cancer researchers is the p53 gene. A mistake, or mutation, in this gene is present in more than 50 percent of all tumors. You'll learn more about the p53 gene, along with the 17 or so other tumor suppressor genes, later in this book.

PROMOTION

For cancer to develop and grow, two events must take place: a change in a gene that affects cell growth, and exposure to something that promotes cell growth. This so-called two-hit theory explains why not all women who inherit a breast cancer gene actually develop breast cancer and why not all smokers get lung cancer.

More than likely, several genetic mutations are necessary to trigger cancer. As scientists continue to discover and map genes, they also will be able to determine which combinations of genetic errors affect a person's cancer risk.

A promoter is something that speeds up the pace of cell division, which can create more genetic mutations and deliver the second hit that leads to cancer. A promoter may be a hormone such as estrogen or a toxic substance such as a chemical in tobacco smoke. Researchers believe that obesity and poor diet may act as promoters, though the mechanisms behind them aren't clear. Some factors, like radiation, can play the dual roles of initiator and promoter.

Fortunately, from a prevention point of view, some substances can interfere with cancer promotion. For instance, certain types of dietary fiber curtail the absorption of carcinogens in the intestine. In laboratory experiments, antioxidants such as vitamins A, C, and E act as anticarcinogens. On the other hand, deficiencies in these nutrients may contribute to certain cancers.

The cancer process still can turn around at the promotion stage, depending on the amount of genetic damage. But scientists don't know for certain when this window of opportunity closes. Until they can answer this question, avoiding promoters remains an important aspect of cancer prevention.

PROGRESSION

The term *progression* refers to the out-of-control growth of abnormal cells that is the basis of all cancers. As explained earlier, the cells accumulate to form a tumor, and the tumor keeps growing, possibly extending into adjacent tissues. In addition, cells may spread to other parts of the body, forming clusters there.

How quickly a cancer progresses is determined in part by genetic programming. It also is influenced by conditions in the body, such as the presence of certain hormones. Even once progression begins, a vigilant immune system still may destroy cancer cells, significantly interfering with the disease process, if not stopping it entirely. Cancer growth may be so slow that the malignant cells never cause a problem. In support of this fact, it's estimated that cancer is present in the organs of 10 to 15 percent of people who die from other causes.

PREVENTION IS PARAMOUNT

Now that you have a basic understanding of what's involved in the cancer process, you can see how prevention could be your best defense against the disease. You have many options for stopping cancer before it gains a foothold. For instance, you can limit your contact with substances that initiate or promote the disease. You can enhance the body's immune defenses and cellular repair systems. Pinpointing and treating precancers offer another avenue of attack. So, too, does turning on or off the various mechanisms that drive cell growth.

Some of these preventive measures are available now. Many more are on the frontier of cancer prevention. We'll explore them in depth in the chapters that follow.

CHAPTER 2

A

STATISTICAL

PERSPECTIVE

• • • • • • • • • •

IN RECENT YEARS, SOME EXPERTS HAVE taken to de-
scribing cancer as an epidemic. And perhaps with good reason, when you
consider that everyone seems to know someone with the disease and that
the number of known cases rises each year. By the end of 2004, more than
1.3 million people could learn that they have cancer. And this doesn't include the million or more with certain types of skin cancer, or those with
early-stage noninvasive cancers. If current estimates hold true, the
number of people facing a cancer diagnosis will double over the next 50
years, to 2.6 million.

Yes, these statistics are frightening. But consider them in the context
of two important facts. First, the U.S. population continues to grow, which
means there are more Americans who could get cancer. Second, the el-
derly segment of the population is growing exceptionally fast, and cancer
is mainly a disease of aging.

Many of the illnesses that once proved fatal at a younger age don't
pose as great a threat today. As a result, we Americans are living longer
than ever. The life expectancy in the United States is at an all-time high—

Age and Cancer

IF YOU ARE AGE . . .	YOUR RISK OF DEVELOPING BREAST CANCER IS 1 IN . . .
20	2,044
30	249
40	67
50	36
60	29
70	24

Source: American Cancer Society, Surveillance Research, 2001

74 years for men, about 80 years for women. The number of Americans over age 75 will triple by the year 2050.

Our increasing longevity means that more of us are living long enough to get cancer. Actually, about 77 percent of all cancers occur in people ages 55 and older. By comparison, childhood cancers are rare, with about 9,200 new cases expected in 2004.

The reality is that when the data are adjusted to eliminate the impact of the rising average age of the population, the rate of cancer in the United States has held steady and even declined slightly over the past few years. Statistically speaking, we've seen little change in cancer incidence or death in the past 40 years.

THE RISE AND FALL OF A DISEASE

It's true that the incidences of certain kinds of cancer have gone through some ups and downs. But the ups are not inexplicable.

Technically, the rise in the number of cases of primary lung cancer, melanoma, and AIDS-related cancers does not qualify as an epidemic. Rather, experts refer to this kind of increase as excessive prevalence, which simply means that a large number of people have a particular disease. To qualify as an epidemic, a disease must occur suddenly and with a frequency clearly in excess of normal expectancy.

Lung cancer once was a rare disease. But the popularity of cigarette smoking, which surged at about the turn of the 20th century and didn't

Speaking Cancer's Language

When you read or hear news reports about cancer, they may use various terms to describe how many people have the disease. Understanding these terms is very important to accurately interpret the statistics in the reports. To this end, the following definitions may come in handy.

INCIDENCE: The number of new cases diagnosed in a particular place over a specific time period, usually a year.

INCIDENCE RATE: The number of new cases diagnosed among a standard number of people—say, 100,000—during a year. It also may refer to the incidence divided by the number of people in a given area.

MORTALITY: The number of people who die from cancer in a particular place over a specific time period, usually a year.

MORTALITY RATE: The number of deaths among a standard number of people during a year. It also may refer to the number of deaths divided by the number of people in a given area.

ADJUSTED: A change in the incidence rate or mortality rate to account for the influence of a specific factor, such as age.

AGE-ADJUSTED RATE: A calculation of the number of people with cancer among a standard number of people of about the same age. When we compare incidence rates or mortality rates, knowing whether or not the figures are age-adjusted is crucial. Otherwise, the rates may appear to be much higher than they actually are.

PREVALENCE: The percentage of people who have cancer, both old and new cases, out of the number who are at risk for it.

drop off until the 1960s, produced a dramatic but nevertheless explainable or expected rise in lung cancer cases over the years. For men, the incidence peaked in the mid-1980s and then declined significantly. For women, the incidence didn't taper off until the 1990s. This is because women took up smoking later, and quit later, than men. The bottom line is, while we did see a spike in the number of people with lung cancer, it was not an epidemic.

Today we're witnessing a jump in the frequency of melanoma, which experts attribute to our penchant for sunbathing. In the 1970s, the incidence of the disease was climbing rapidly, by about 6 percent per year. But since the 1980s, the rate of increase has slowed to about 3 percent per year.

Also in the 1980s, we saw a rise in the prevalence of HIV (human immunodeficiency virus) infection. This led to a corresponding increase in HIV-related cancers such as non-Hodgkin's lymphoma, multiple myeloma, and Kaposi's sarcoma, especially in younger people.

WHAT THE NUMBERS REALLY MEAN

Without question, the persistently high prevalence of cancer in the U.S. population is a major public health issue. But statistics about the disease can be more alarming than necessary, depending on how they are presented.

For instance, in our introduction to this book, we mentioned that cancer soon will replace heart disease as the number one cause of death in the United States. This is true. But cancer is moving to the top position *not* because of a dramatic increase in the disease—which would qualify as an epidemic—or even because of a gradual rise in the number of people diagnosed with or dying from it. Rather, cancer will assume the number one spot because the death rate from heart disease is declining. This is happening for several reasons. First, the number of Americans who develop heart disease has dropped significantly. Second, care and treatment for heart disease has improved. Third, fewer Americans are smoking, a habit that raises the risk of both heart disease and cancer.

The way the media interpret the odds of getting cancer tends to fuel public fears about the disease. Again, putting these statistics into proper perspective makes them less ominous. As an example, you might hear that a man has a one-in-two chance of developing cancer in his lifetime, and a woman, a one-in-three chance. Although this may seem like an epidemic, remember what we said earlier about cancer's being a disease of aging? These statistics represent lifetime risk—that is, your chances of getting cancer over your entire life span. And as you now know, that risk increases with age. Cancer is 100 times more common among men at age 75 than at age 25. For women, the later years bring a 30-times-greater risk of the disease.

The statistics about breast cancer can be especially frightening. It's true that breast cancer accounts for nearly one in every three cancers among women. It also is true that breast cancer ranks second only to lung cancer in cancer deaths among women. But with breast cancer, as with most other malignancies, the incidence increases with age. In fact, 77 percent of new breast cancer cases occur in those ages 50 and older. We don't mean to imply that women needn't be concerned about the disease. But the United States is not experiencing a breast cancer epidemic, as some news reports might suggest.

When University of Michigan researchers conducted an analysis of more than 200 articles published in the late 1980s and the 1990s, they noticed that the articles failed to establish a connection between the rise in breast cancer cases and improvements in early detection through greater use of mammography. Rather, the articles portrayed the 27.2 percent increase as " . . . a mysterious, unexplained epidemic occurring primarily among young, professional women in their prime years." The fact is, the increase was anything but mysterious. And it slowed in the 1990s as the use of mammography reached a plateau.

With any cancer, a rise in the number of cases may reflect improvements in screening methods or diagnostic testing. For example, when CT scans became available, doctors could more easily detect tumors in the central nervous system, which led to an increase in the number of diagnosed brain tumors. Similarly, the development of the prostate-specific antigen (PSA) test, which checks the blood for a marker of prostate cancer, and greater use of the digital rectal exam led to more frequent diagnosis of prostate cancer in men. But after the discovery of all those early-stage cancers between 1992 and 1995, the incidence of prostate cancer fell dramatically and has since reached a plateau.

Even the so-called epidemic of environmentally caused cancers in the 1970s, which coincided with the creation of the Environmental Protection Agency, was determined to have never existed a decade later. Studies showed that no more than 3 percent of cancers result from chemicals in the environment, rather than the 70 to 90 percent figure tossed about at the height of the scare. Again, this doesn't mean that we shouldn't be concerned about the health hazards of pollution. But we should be realistic in our appraisal of environmental risk.

CHAPTER 3

UNDERSTANDING

RISK

* * * * *

SOME 300 YEARS HAVE PASSED since scientists first realized that cancer is associated with certain aspects of a person's life—what we now refer to as risk factors. Back then, breast cancer appeared more commonly in celibate nuns. The scientists attributed this pattern to the fact that the nuns had never been pregnant. Modern research has confirmed that when women never experience pregnancy—a risk factor called nulliparity—they are continually exposed to the hormone estrogen, which increases their likelihood of developing breast cancer. In fact, we know for certain that becoming pregnant at an early age is one natural way to reduce lifetime breast cancer risk. Breastfeeding is another.

Some risk factors are part of our genetic programming and therefore beyond our control, such as the age at which we begin puberty or go through menopause. Age itself is among the most significant indicators of cancer risk.

But many other risk factors are within our control—especially those behaviors, or lifestyle factors, that we change by choice. Smokers who decide to quit, for example, lower their chances of developing lung cancer. Similarly, people who take steps to shield their skin from the sun are less susceptible to skin cancer, including melanoma. And limiting alcohol consumption appears to lower the risk of liver cancer.

Several large epidemiologic studies have offered convincing proof that lifestyle factors can influence cancer risk for better or for worse. Research has found, for instance, that Japanese women have a much lower rate of breast cancer than their American counterparts. But when they move to the United States and adopt a higher-fat Western diet, their risk of breast cancer rises to equal that of American women within 5 years. Other studies show that second-generation Japanese-Americans have a higher incidence of colorectal cancer than Japanese who remain in their native country.

Some risk factors for cancer carry more weight than others. The presence of multiple risk factors is significant, too. But it doesn't mean that cancer is a certainty. By the same token, having no risk factors doesn't mean that a person never will get cancer. Still, one of the most important measures in cancer prevention is to change or minimize any risk factors that are within our control.

According to the American Cancer Society, the majority of cancers are preventable. Reducing risk means giving up unhealthy habits like smoking, and adopting healthy behaviors like engaging in regular physical activity and eating more fruits and vegetables. It also involves the early detection and treatment of conditions that could lead to cancer.

Another important aspect of cancer prevention is knowing your genetic risk. True, you can't reshuffle the genetic cards you're dealt at birth. But by being aware of your family history, you might become even more vigilant about managing the lifestyle factors that influence your cancer risk and getting regular screening tests. You also can talk with your doctor about additional testing that isn't routine for people who don't have strong family histories of particular cancers, but that might be helpful for you. You'll learn more about these specialized screening tests in chapter 4, as well as in the cancer-specific chapters in part 2.

GENETICS VERSUS HEREDITY

Just as genes carry messages about hair and eye color, stature, and skin tone from parent to child, they also can carry susceptibility to cancer.

Some cancers seem to occur in clusters within families, though about 90 percent are sporadic, meaning they have no known hereditary link.

It has been said that all cancers are genetic, but few are inherited. In other words, while all types of cancer result from mistakes in genes, the mistakes haven't necessarily passed from one generation to the next. As we discussed in chapter 1, the genetic mutations that set the stage for cancer can occur spontaneously—triggered by something in the environment, for example, or by cells multiplying faster than normal. These are known as somatic mutations because they can affect any of the body's cells.

Only errors in the genes of the sex cells—that is, the sperm and the eggs, also called germ cells—can pass from parent to child. These are known as germ line mutations. Only germ line mutations in specific genes cause hereditary cancers. For instance, about 1 percent of people with colorectal cancer carry the gene for familial adenomatous polyposis (FAP), in which thousands of polyps form in the colon. FAP leads to cancer in about 95 percent of those who inherit the genetic mutation. Hereditary nonpolyposis colorectal cancer (HNPCC) is another colorectal cancer syndrome, and the most common. Between 70 and 82 percent of those who inherit the genetic mutation associated with HNPCC develop colorectal cancer by age 70. HNPCC also may contribute to cancers outside the colon. For example, women who inherit this genetic mutation have a 42 to 60 percent lifetime risk of endometrial cancer.

Since 25 percent of people—one in four—get cancer sometime in their lives, families who don't have the disease somewhere in their histories are few and far between. In fact, between 10 and 15 percent of cancers are familial.

An inherited cancer may occur among a person's first-degree relatives—the immediate family, including parents, siblings, and children—or among second-degree relatives, such as grandparents, aunts, and uncles. Someone whose mother and uncle or father and aunt are diagnosed with a particular kind of cancer is at higher risk for the disease than someone whose immediate family is cancer-free. A person with a family history of melanoma may have eight times the average risk of developing this most serious form of skin cancer. Similarly, a man whose father, brother, or son develops prostate cancer has double the risk of getting it, too.

Cancer in the Family

Identifying a cancer syndrome such as hereditary nonpolyposis colorectal cancer (HNPCC) requires a careful evaluation of family history. It's helpful, thought not always possible, to obtain reports on the pathology of the cancer that has been diagnosed in a relative. It's also helpful for that person to undergo genetic testing because the test can identify the specific genetic mutation if the cancer is an inherited one. But the first step always should be getting a complete family history.

Here's an example of the family tree of Sarah, a middle-aged woman who was diagnosed with HNPCC while in her thirties.

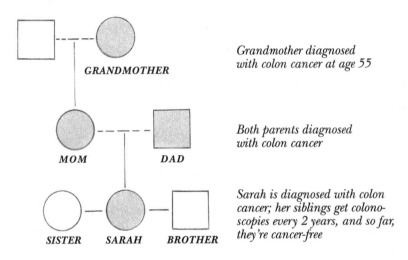

GRANDMOTHER

Grandmother diagnosed with colon cancer at age 55

MOM   DAD

Both parents diagnosed with colon cancer

SISTER   SARAH   BROTHER

Sarah is diagnosed with colon cancer; her siblings get colonoscopies every 2 years, and so far, they're cancer-free

With the above illustration as a model, draw at least three generations of your own family tree, beginning with you and your siblings and tracing back to your grandparents. Use squares to indicate men and circles to represent women. Color in the shape for each relative who's developed cancer, and put a diagonal slash through it if that person has died. Next to each shaded shape, write down what kind of cancer was involved, where it started, and how old the person was when he or she was diagnosed. If the person has died, also make note of the age and cause of death. Keep this family tree with your medical records, along with any copies of pathology reports and genetic test results that you can obtain.

For each of the cancers presented in part 2, you will find a list of questions to help assess your personal risk. In general, you're more likely to inherit cancer if any of the following apply:

- Two or more close relatives have a particular kind of cancer.
- A family member has several primary cancers.
- A family member developed cancer at an early age.
- A family member has a cancer with a known genetic link.

Just as with other risk factors, carrying the genetic blueprint for a certain cancer doesn't mean that you can't avoid the disease. As we noted in chapter 1, more than one genetic mutation—perhaps resulting from a lifestyle factor, such as smoking or a high-fat diet—usually is necessary to launch the cancer process. So although family history plays a key role, and a bigger role in some cancers than in others, it is not the only risk factor. This means you can take steps to to prevent the disease, even when it runs in your family.

IDENTIFYING THE ROGUE GENES

In 1998, the National Cancer Institute founded the Cancer Genetics Network to investigate the genetics of individual susceptibility to cancer and to integrate this new information into medical practice. Thus far, researchers have identified several cancer genes, including BRCA1, BRCA2, and HNPCC. The BRCAs are tumor suppressor genes; any damage to them can raise a woman's risk of breast and ovarian cancers. For example, a woman who inherits one copy of a mutated BRCA1 gene has a 59 percent chance of developing breast cancer by age 50. In part 2 of this book, we'll say more about the various genes that influence the risk of particular cancers.

Some tests for the genetic mutations associated with certain cancers already are available, and more are in the pipeline. The tests don't actually detect cancer; they only identify mutations that could increase risk. Furthermore, not all mutations necessarily lead to cancer.

The testing itself is as simple as providing a blood sample. Deciding to get the test is the hard part, which is why we strongly recommend consulting a knowledgeable physician or a genetic counselor before making up your mind.

Finding out that you carry a genetic mutation that dramatically increases your risk of a particular cancer can be upsetting. But it also can be empowering as you become more proactive about taking the necessary preventive steps—whether they're lifestyle changes, medication, or surgery.

A good example of how awareness affects behavior comes from a recent study that set out to determine who gets routine colonoscopy, a visual examination of the colon and rectum through an endoscope. According to the study findings, people who knew they carried the HNPCC gene mutations associated with colorectal cancer were significantly more likely to undergo screening than those who lacked the mutations. By various estimates, somewhere between 43 and 76 percent of people who are at high risk for colorectal cancer undergo genetic testing.

Detecting a genetic mutation also raises the possibility of entering a clinical trial that is examining a particular chemopreventive drug. Your physician or genetic counselor can help identify your options.

For some people, no preventive measure—not even surgery—is too drastic if it allays the anxiety of knowing that they're highly susceptible to cancer. Let's say a woman carries a BRCA1 or BRCA2 gene mutation, which means that she's three to seven times more likely to develop breast cancer than a woman who doesn't have the mutation. She may decide to improve her odds of avoiding the disease by undergoing the surgical removal of both her breasts. Preventive, or prophylactic, mastectomy does reduce breast cancer risk to about 10 percent. This payoff is worth the sacrifice for some women. Prophylactic oophorectomy, the surgical removal of the ovaries, lowers breast cancer risk by about two-thirds.

A woman who is at risk for ovarian cancer also may opt for prophylactic oophorectomy. This is controversial because the surgery works best when performed before menopause. In effect, it induces menopause, which brings its own discomforts and concerns. Studies have shown that

Checking Your Genes

Researchers have identified genes for several cancers that tend to run in families. So far, genetic testing is available for the following:

- Breast cancer
- Familial adenomatous polyposis (FAP)
- Familial medullary thyroid carcinoma (FMTC)
- Hereditary nonpolyposis colon cancer (HNPCC)
- Li-Fraumeni syndrome
- Ovarian cancer
- Retinoblastoma and Wilms' tumor

If your family's history includes any of these cancers, you may want to consult a genetic counselor to determine whether you're a candidate for testing. Keep in mind that only 10 to 15 percent of cancers are familial.

while prophylactic oophorectomy significantly lowers ovarian cancer risk, it doesn't entirely eliminate it.

In a Canadian study of 75 women who underwent surgical removal of both breasts because of concerns about developing breast cancer, researchers determined that perceived cancer risk was much higher than actual risk. The study participants had completed a questionnaire in which they estimated their chances of developing cancer at 76.2 percent, on average. Even among those who carried the breast cancer gene, their risk was notably lower than they thought—about 59 percent. And some didn't even have the genetic mutation, so their risk was lower still.

We'll say more about surgery as a preventive measure in chapters 9 and 12, which address breast and ovarian cancers respectively. For now, these study findings highlight why genetic counseling is so important for anyone who's susceptible to an inherited cancer. A physician or counselor can help accurately assess individual risk through family history and possibly genetic testing.

YOUR PERSONAL RISK PROFILE

Now that we've explored the big picture of cancer risk, let's apply it to you personally. What are the odds that you will develop cancer in the next decade? In the next two or three?

Not all cancers share the same set of risk factors. And as we mentioned earlier, some risk factors—primarily those involving lifestyle choices—are amenable to change, while others are immutable. The "givens" include age, gender, and race and ethnicity, all of which we'll discuss in further detail here.

AGE. You've already learned that the most influential of all cancer risk factors is age. No one knows for sure why this is so, though scientists offer some credible theories. One is that when you're young, you have healthy, active immune cells that can ferret out and destroy abnormal cells before they cause cancer. But your immune system becomes weaker over time, and your immune cells don't perform their jobs as well. The repair mechanisms that correct mistakes in our genes may falter, too.

We believe this theory to be true based on our clinical experience with patients who have illnesses that weaken the immune system, such as HIV infection, or who take immunity-suppressing medications. They tend to develop cancer much more readily than healthy people, regardless of age.

Another reason that age may raise cancer risk is that the damage from certain substances builds up over years of exposure to them. It may take a certain amount of cumulative damage to tip the balance between genetic injury and repair in favor of cancer.

GENDER. Prostate cancer is the most common form of cancer in men, while breast cancer takes the top spot for women. Obviously, women won't get prostate cancer because they lack prostate glands. And men seldom develop breast cancer because they have little glandular tissue in their breasts and a minute supply of estrogen.

Beyond cancers that affect the reproductive organs, the risk of other cancers seems about equal for men and women. Lung cancer is the second most common cancer in both genders; colorectal cancer ranks third.

The ebb and flow of hormones changes with age and, for women, with the various reproductive stages. In part 2, you'll learn how certain hormones can influence the risk of specific cancers. For now, keep in mind that you can manipulate levels of some hormones to improve your odds of staying cancer-free. For instance, women may choose to take oral contraceptives to help protect against ovarian cancer. The Pill may help for several reasons. First, a woman who's taking oral contraceptives doesn't ovulate, and this "break" may provide a protective effect. Second, hormones may be less stimulating in the presence of the Pill. And third, hormones called progestins in oral contraceptives may encourage normal ovarian cell death. The effect of estrogen from many sources on the occurrence of cancer in women is an active area of scientific research.

RACE AND ETHNICITY. In examining the impact of race and ethnicity on cancer risk, scientists have struggled to separate socioeconomic factors from the mix. Nevertheless, some studies have made a point of accounting for the roles of education and income in access to health care—all of which help determine who gets cancer and who doesn't. By matching groups of Whites with groups from other races, all sharing similar educational backgrounds and income levels, researchers have made headway in understanding race and ethnicity as cancer risk factors.

For reasons not yet understood, Whites have higher rates of most cancers than any other racial group in the United States. The exceptions to this "rule" are cancers of the cervix, prostate, and pancreas, which tend to occur more often in African-Americans. For example, the incidence of prostate cancer is 60 percent higher in African-American men than in White men. In fact, prostate cancer is the most common cancer among African-American men.

Until 1997, the incidence of cancer among African-Americans had been on the rise, significantly so. But now that steady climb is diminishing at a rate of about 2.5 percent per year. Deaths from cancer among African-Americans have declined substantially in the past decade as well, though the death rate remains higher than for Whites. In fact, the gap between the two groups is larger now than in 1975.

In general, the incidence of cancer is lower among Hispanics than among White non-Hispanics, and is declining ever more quickly. Breast cancer is the most common cancer among Hispanic women, while prostate cancer is the most common among Hispanic men.

African-Americans and Cancer

Among all racial and ethnic groups, African-Americans are the most likely to die from cancer. While the incidence of the disease is 20 percent higher among African-American men than among White men, the death rate is 40 percent higher. African-Americans of both genders are 60 percent more likely to develop cancer than Hispanics, and twice as likely as Native Americans.

An estimated 132,700 African-Americans were diagnosed with cancer in 2003. In this population, the incidence of the disease peaked in 1993, and has been dropping ever since—on average, about 2.5 percent per year. Likewise, the death rate has declined by about 1.1 percent per year. These statistics reflect a definite improvement from the early 1990s, although African-Americans continue to show a shorter survival time than Whites, regardless of when they develop cancer.

Among African-American men, the most common cancers are prostate, lung, and colon and rectum. African-American women are most vulnerable to breast cancer, followed by cancers of the colon and rectum and of the lung. In fact, the incidence of breast cancer is higher in African-American women than in White women prior to age 40. Beyond age 40, White women are more likely to develop the disease.

After years of increases, the death rate from breast cancer among African-American women finally has begun to plateau. Among women under age 50, it already is dropping off. Nevertheless, it remains higher than for White women. Researchers offer several explanations for this phenomenon. One is that African-American women receive their diagnoses at more advanced stages. Another is that they may have more aggressive, faster-growing forms of breast cancer.

The incidence of prostate cancer is about 60 percent higher in African-American men than in White men. The incidence seemed to peak in the late 1980s and early 1990s because of the increased use of prostate-specific antigen (PSA) testing. Though prostate cancer remains the second leading cause of cancer death among African-American men, the death rate is declining, for reasons that scientists cannot yet explain.

Hispanic Americans and Cancer

Compared with Whites who are not of Hispanic descent, Hispanic Americans have a lower incidence of virtually all cancers except those of the stomach, liver, and cervix. The most common cancers among people in this ethnic group are those of the breast, prostate, lung, and colon and rectum—which also happen to be the most common among non-Hispanic Whites.

The incidence of cervical cancer is twice as high in Hispanic women as in women of other ethnic backgrounds, perhaps because of inadequate Pap testing. In addition, Hispanic women tend to be diagnosed at a more advanced stage of the disease, which may help explain why the death rate from cervical cancer is 40 percent higher for them than for non-Hispanic women.

In the 1990s, the rate of breast cancer declined among Hispanic women, while it continued to rise among Whites. Still, Hispanic women receive their diagnoses later in life, perhaps because they're less likely to get mammograms. As with cervical cancer, breast cancer in Hispanic women usually is more advanced by the time it's caught.

As with African-American and White men, prostate cancer is the most common among Hispanic men. But their cancer rate is about 20 percent lower than those of the other ethnic groups.

Several inherited diseases—such as Tay-Sachs disease and type 1 Gaucher disease, as well as breast, ovarian, and colon cancers—are common among descendants of the Ashkenazi Jews, who lived in eastern or central Europe a half century ago. Back then, these people lived in relative isolation and married within their groups, passing on certain genetic errors to their offspring. Today about 80 percent of ethnic Jews in the United States are of Ashkenazi descent.

In 1995, researchers determined that 1 percent of the Jewish population carry a mutation in the BRCA1 breast cancer gene. By comparison, only about 0.1 to 0.6 percent of all Americans have this mutated gene. Further study found that another mutation in BRCA1, as well as a mutation in BRCA2, is more likely to occur in Ashkenazi Jews. If you're of this heritage, you have a 2.3 percent chance of carrying one of these mutations.

The first report from the Molecular Epidemiology of Colorectal Cancer Study, a collaborative effort between the United States and Israel, found that people of Ashkenazi descent are two to three times more likely to develop colorectal cancer. Inheriting mutations in what's known as the BLM gene from one parent could increase risk significantly. Colorectal cancer is the leading cause of cancer deaths in Israel.

Just recently, scientists have begun to investigate the incidences of certain cancers in Asian-Americans. Just as Hispanics differ according to their nation of origin, Asians come from China, Japan, Korea, Thailand, and many other countries and encompass more than 30 distinct ethnic groups. In general, Asian-Americans have a relatively low cancer risk, but compared with other ethnic groups, their death rate from the disease appears to be rising more quickly. Asian-Americans and Pacific Islanders are three times more likely than Whites to die from liver cancer, and twice as likely to die from stomach cancer. In addition, cervical cancer is five times more common in Asian-American women than in White women.

THE ODDS OF RECURRENCE

Having cancer once increases your chances of getting it again. Cancer cells from the original tumor may spread to create a secondary cancer at another site. Or an entirely new cancer may develop in association with the same risk factors that contributed to the initial malignancy. For instance, a smoker who managed to beat lung cancer remains at risk for throat cancer. On rare occasions, a new cancer totally unrelated to the prior one can occur.

Prevention may be more important for cancer survivors than for anyone else. Whether they beat the disease long ago or they're in the thick of the battle, taking steps to minimize the chances of a recurrence is an essential component of treatment. Cancer survivors should continue to get screening tests to catch any abnormalities early on. Depending on the type of cancer, their doctors may recommend more frequent testing than usual. These people also may have periodic tests to monitor those organs most likely to be affected by a secondary cancer. For instance, a person with colorectal cancer may undergo testing of liver function at established intervals.

Another active area of scientific research involves tests to identify particular indicators, or biomarkers, that may help predict whether a cancer is likely to recur or spread, initiating a secondary cancer. We're especially optimistic about a test called DNA microarray analysis, which involves the examination of hundreds of genes from the DNA of a person's cancer cells for characteristic clues about a cancer's aggressiveness.

The test results may tell us, for example, whether a woman who has been treated for breast cancer would benefit from chemopreventive therapy with tamoxifen. We'll say more about specific tests, and the clinical trials to evaluate their usefulness, later in this book.

PERCEPTION ISN'T REALITY

How concerned you are about cancer has a lot to do with how much control you have over your risk. *New York Times* health columnist Jane Brody wrote about an acquaintance who participates in dangerous sports like rock climbing and white-water rafting, yet eats only organically grown food. The woman's extreme activities, Brody noted, are "far riskier than all the chemical fertilizers, pesticides, and antibiotics combined." All of us have known people like this—people who are overly cautious, if not phobic, about some aspect of life when other aspects present far greater dangers, statistically speaking. Perhaps we're this way ourselves.

What makes one woman fearful of food but not of heights, or terrified of flying but not of driving on the freeway, is that she believes she has more control in one situation than the other. Whether it involves being tethered to the side of a mountain or changing lanes, a sense of being in control tends to diminish fear.

A family history of cancer is one of those things that we can't choose. So those of us who are at high risk may respond in extreme and opposing ways. Some assume that they will get cancer no matter what, resign them-selves to their fate, and do little to lower their chances. They may even avoid screening tests that could detect cancerous changes early on. Others are at the opposite end of the spectrum, interpreting every twinge as a sign of cancer.

Between these two extremes is the woman who says, "Since my mother died from colorectal cancer at age 43, my risk is higher than my husband's, whose parents are alive and well at 70. So I'm going to do whatever I can to lower my risk. And I'm going to have routine screening tests earlier and maybe more often than my husband does." Depending on the type of cancer, this woman may want to consider testing to deter-mine whether she carries a genetic mutation that could increase her risk.

Women routinely overestimate their chances of developing breast cancer. The reality is, the average 40-year-old woman who has never smoked has only a 0.2 percent chance of dying from breast cancer by the time she turns 50. According to a Dartmouth University researcher who studies risk perception, we can't accurately assess our personal risk if we have nothing against which to gauge the statistics. And for some of us, those statistics loom frighteningly large, obscuring other, perhaps more dangerous risk factors.

As an example, let's suppose that same 40-year-old woman does smoke, which means she has a 13 percent chance of dying from lung cancer by age 70. She may be worried about getting breast cancer, but her chances of getting lung cancer are far higher.

A realistic awareness of your cancer risk is essential to cancer pre-vention because it affects almost every decision, from which screening tests to have to which lifestyle changes to make. If you are at high risk, your choices may include trying a chemopreventive therapy or enrolling in a clinical trial to evaluate such a therapy. If you are at very high risk, you may want to look into options such as genetic testing, prophylactic surgery, or special diagnostic tests.

CHAPTER 4

SCREENING

• • • • • • • • • • •

Between reminders from your doctor and public service announcements on radio and TV, you probably have gotten the message that when it comes to cancer, early detection increases the chances of cure. Screening tests for cancers of the breast, cervix, prostate, testes, colon and rectum, mouth and throat, and skin are widely available and in regular use. In fact, the American Cancer Society states that if all Americans got these screenings in accordance with established guidelines, the 5-year survival rate for the corresponding cancers would increase by 15 percent.

Sometimes detectable precancerous changes appear long before cancer actually occurs. If these early changes are identified and treated, the cancer may be prevented entirely.

You may think of screening tests such as the Pap test (which samples cells from the surface of the cervix) and the fecal occult blood test (which checks for blood in the stool, a possible sign of precancerous intestinal polyps) as tools for cancer detection. And they are. By definition, screening tests are performed on healthy people to look for cancer that has not produced noticeable symptoms, in what is known as the detectable preclinical phase. But some screening tests also can pick up cancer precursors—that is, conditions that precede cancer. For example, screening tests of the cervix and the colon and rectum are for the primary purpose of detecting cancer precursors. When used in this capacity, screening tests are considered a secondary preventive measure.

Sometimes you may hear precursors described as precancers. This is because such lesions are highly likely to become cancers. A good example of a precancer is a leukoplakia, a reddish or whitish patch of abnormal cells. A leukoplakia might appear in a smoker's mouth, inside the cheek or on the tongue.

You may not realize it, but your dentist is looking for precancers when he shines a bright light inside your cheeks and along your gum line and asks that you move your tongue this way and that. Examining the entire inside of your mouth for white or red patches and checking for other abnormalities, like difficulty swallowing, should be part of every routine dental exam. (If you want to be sure that your dentist is doing this, ask if he is checking for spots that could be precancers.)

If a screening test finds a lesion, and examination of the cells indicates that the lesion is in the process of becoming a cancer, it can be treated with medication or surgery, or possibly with a chemopreventive agent. For instance, research has shown that topical retinoids may keep a leukoplakia from turning malignant, though they aren't in wide use for this purpose.

One difference between a cancer precursor and an early cancer is that a precursor may not become a cancer. In fact, some naturally regress. This is why cancer experts continue to debate what treatment, if any, should follow the detection of certain precursors. You may encounter this dilemma if you must choose between treating a potentially precancerous condition and taking a "watch and wait" approach to see if the condition actually progresses to cancer. Choosing to watch and wait means you will need more frequent checkups to monitor the abnormality. In part 2, we will provide the most current information about cancer precursors so you can make an informed decision about whether and how you should respond if you're found to have one.

STOPPING CANCER BEFORE IT STARTS

Thanks to advances in molecular biology, scientists are finding new ways to detect cellular changes at their earliest stages, before they lead to cancer. They also are developing new tools and techniques to retrieve cells from all parts of the body, without surgery or pain. One such technique, which we'll explain in more detail in chapter 9, allows a physician to obtain cells from within the breast ducts with minimal discomfort. Analysis of these cells can reveal whether abnormalities that could progress to cancer are occurring within the ducts, where most breast cancer begins. This test is especially useful for women who are at high risk for the disease.

Other tests look for certain cancer biomarkers in the bloodstream. These substances, which come from cells, indicate that the cancer process already has begun. For example, the presence of a protein called CA-125 is a red flag for ovarian cancer. Similarly, large amounts of prostate-specific antigen (PSA)—which is produced by cells in the prostate gland and is found in semen—may point to an abnormal condition in the prostate, including cancer.

Over time, scientists will identify even more substances that could alert both physician and patient to precancerous changes. For a physician, the presence of such a biomarker would serve as a cue to investigate further. For the patient, the awareness of increased cancer risk may prompt extra vigilance, in terms of more frequent checkups or screenings, or perhaps chemopreventive therapy. Scientists also are investigating whether measurable changes in DNA, a shift in the rate of cell division or growth, or alterations to substances that stimulate cell growth could be detectable biomarkers for precancers.

While screening tests are for healthy people at all levels of risk, the frequency of testing may vary with the severity of risk. Some tests are best reserved for those who are most likely to develop certain kinds of cancer. Others are genetic tests, intended to assess a person's cancer susceptibility. We'll say more about these in part 2, when we talk about specific cancers.

WHERE SCREENING GUIDELINES COME FROM

Many government agencies, medical societies, and health organizations have established guidelines for cancer screening tests. These groups base their recommendations on thorough evaluations of the scientific evidence regarding the safety and accuracy of the tests, the sensitivity of the tests in detecting cancer and cancer precursors, the cost of providing tests to those who need them, and the benefit of knowing the results.

For various reasons, the groups don't always agree. And like any institution, each is subject to outside pressures of one sort or another. One particular concern is cost, especially in countries that have single-payer health care systems, like Canada. In the United States, where the government doesn't regulate health care, recommendations—particularly for tests to detect cancer precursors—tend to be more liberal. Still, whether the testing is covered by insurance companies and managed care plans can vary considerably.

The U.S. Preventive Services Task Force (USPSTF) is the government agency that makes recommendations for public health care policy, including preventive services such as immunizations and cancer screening tests. The USPSTF assigns letter grades from A to E to their recommendations for screening tests, based on the scientific evidence in support of each test. For instance, both the Pap test and mammography earn an A for women between ages 50 and 69. In the USPSTF's words, "There is good evidence to support the recommendation (that the condition) be specifically considered in a periodic health examination." On the other hand, the chest x-ray and the PSA test get a D, meaning "there is fair evidence to support the recommendation that the condition be excluded from consideration in a periodic health examination." In fact, the USPSTF recently concluded that there is not sufficient evidence to recommend for or against routine screening for prostate cancer.

Another source of guidelines for screening tests is the National Cancer Institute, which bases its recommendations on the Physician Data Query database program. This program continually reviews scientific studies and recommendations by other institutions and periodically releases statements about cancer screening and early detection.

AMERICAN CANCER SOCIETY GUIDELINES

Many experts consider the American Cancer Society's recommendations to be the gold standard among screening guidelines. For this reason, we've chosen to include them here. You'll find more detailed explanations of various tests and exams in part 2, where we discuss the nine most common cancers. Those chapters also will identify screening tests that may not be appropriate for everyone but that could be helpful for people at high risk for certain cancers.

CANCER-RELATED CHECKUP

The ACS recommends a cancer-related checkup every 3 years for people between ages 20 and 40, and every year for people ages 40 and older. This exam should include health counseling and—depending on someone's age—examinations for cancers of the thyroid, oral cavity, skin, lymph nodes, testes, and ovaries, as well as for some nonmalignant diseases.

BREAST

Physicians should inform their female patients about the benefits and limitations of monthly breast self-exam. These guidelines also apply.

- Clinical physical breast examination every 3 years for women ages 20 to 40 and every year after age 40; this exam should occur close to, and ideally before, a scheduled mammogram
- Mammography every year for women ages 40 and over

CERVIX

A woman should begin cervical cancer screening within 3 years of first engaging in vaginal intercourse, but no later than age 21. Screening should occur every year with the regular Pap test or every 2 years with the newer, liquid-based Pap test. At or after age 30, women who get normal results for three tests in a row may cut back on their screenings to every 2 to 3 years. Those ages 70 and older who get normal results on at least three consecutive tests, and who've had no abnormal results for at least 10 years, may choose to discontinue screenings altogether.

A doctor may recommend more frequent Pap tests if a woman has certain risk factors, such as human immunodeficiency virus (HIV) infection or a weakened immune system. Screening after a total hysterectomy (removal of the uterus and cervix) is not necessary unless the procedure is a treatment for cervical cancer or a precancer. Other special circumstances may require ongoing screening as well. For example, women who've undergone hysterectomy without removal of the cervix should continue with screenings at least until age 70.

COLON AND RECTUM

Beginning at age 50, both men and women of average cancer risk should choose one of the following five testing schedules:

- Fecal occult blood test every year, using a home testing kit for multiple stool samples
- Flexible sigmoidoscopy every 5 years
- Fecal occult blood test every year plus flexible sigmoidoscopy every 5 years; this combination is preferred over either test alone
- Double-contrast barium enema every 5 years
- Colonoscopy every 10 years, or after positive results on any of the previous tests

People should begin colorectal cancer screening earlier and/or undergo screening more often if they have any of these risk factors:

- A personal history of colorectal cancer or adenomatous polyps
- A strong family history of colorectal cancer or polyps, as indicated by either condition in a first-degree relative before age 60 or in two first-degree relatives of any age (remember that a first-degree relative is a parent, sibling, or child)
- A personal history of chronic inflammatory bowel disease
- A family history of a hereditary colorectal cancer syndrome (familial adenomatous polyposis or hereditary nonpolyposis colon cancer)

ENDOMETRIUM

All women should be informed about the risks and symptoms of endometrial cancer and strongly encouraged to report any unexpected bleeding or spotting to their doctors. Those with or at high risk for

hereditary nonpolyposis colon cancer should be given the option of annual screening for endometrial cancer with endometrial biopsy beginning at age 35.

PROSTATE

The death rate from prostate cancer has declined, but whether it's a direct result of screening is not known for certain. For this reason, the ACS
advises physicians to educate their male patients about the potential benefits and risks of early detection and treatment for prostate cancer. In addition, they should offer both prostate-specific antigen (PSA) testing and
digital rectal examination (DRE) to men with a life expectancy of at least
10 years, beginning at age 50.

Men who choose to undergo testing should start at age 50. The exceptions are those in high-risk groups, such as African-American men and
men with a first-degree relative who developed prostate cancer while
young; they should begin testing at age 45. According to the ACS guidelines, doctors should not discourage prostate cancer screening for any patient. If a man asks his doctor to make a decision about screening on his
behalf, the doctor should recommend both the PSA test and DRE.

In men who show no symptoms of prostate cancer, testing can detect
tumors at a more favorable stage. For the PSA test, an abnormal result is
a value above 4.0 ng/ml (nanograms per milliliter). Keep in mind,
though, that elevated PSA can result not only from cancer but also from
benign prostate conditions.

Compared with the PSA test, the digital rectal exam is less effective
in detecting prostate cancer. For best results, DRE should be performed
by a skilled health care professional who can recognize subtle prostate abnormalities.

OTHER GROUPS WEIGH IN

Organizations that represent various medical specialties also offer
screening guidelines for those cancers that their doctors may diagnose
and treat. For example, the American College of Obstetricians and Gynecologists (ACOG) endorses a screening schedule for cervical cancer

that differs from American Cancer Society recommendations. According to the ACOG guidelines, women should get their first Pap test approximately 3 years after beginning sexual intercourse or by age 21, whichever occurs first. The screening should continue on an annual basis up to age 30. At that point, a woman who has gotten negative results on at least three consecutive tests can reduce her screenings from every year to every 2 or 3 years.

Women ages 30 and older also may opt for a Pap test and a test for certain types of human papillomavirus (HPV) that are known risk factors for cervical cancer. If they get negative results on both tests, they require screening only every 3 years. More frequent screening may be necessary if either test comes back positive.

Another example of possible variations in screening guidelines pertains to early detection of skin cancer. The American Academy of Dermatology suggests an annual exam, while the ACS makes no specific recommendation for skin screening.

In part 2, when we turn our attention to specific cancers, we will point out where the ACS guidelines differ from other organizations' recommendations and explain the issues that may be driving these differences. Then you and your doctor can use this information to establish a screening schedule that reflects your unique risk factors and health concerns.

A SCREENING SCHEDULE THAT SUITS YOU

This brings us to an important point: All of the guidelines presented above apply to the general population. They may need some adjustment to fit your particular situation. This is why we recommend working closely with your physician to customize a screening schedule just for you. Your physician can evaluate your family history, as well as certain lifestyle factors that may affect the frequency of screenings. She also will consider your personal medical history, which is why you need to keep good records not just of illnesses and procedures but also of previous test results. Depending on your personal risk profile, your doctor may suggest adding other tests to your screening schedule.

On page 272, you'll find a chart of screening tests organized by age, based on the ACS screening guidelines. We suggest taking this chart to your next doctor's appointment and reviewing it with your doctor. The two of you may decide to modify the age at which you begin certain screenings, or the intervals at which you repeat them. Make a copy of the chart and post it on your refrigerator or put it in your daily planner so you won't forget what tests you need and when.

CHAPTER 5

PREVENTION

. . . .

SINCE WE'RE GYNECOLOGISTS, WOMEN COME to us when they are healthy, as well as when they're sick. Perhaps they need to have a checkup or to talk about birth control. Maybe they are trying to become pregnant and finding it difficult. Or they're approaching menopause and want to be fully informed on what to expect. Of course, if they come because they are experiencing troublesome symptoms, we do the necessary exams, pinpoint the problem and its cause, and suggest an appropriate treatment. But whether our patients are sick or well, some aspect of cancer prevention is integral to every visit.

We may tell a woman who is getting older and beginning to gain weight that she needs to start trimming the fat from her diet and, just as important, to watch her portion sizes as a means of cutting calories. We may encourage a busy career woman to schedule appointments with herself for exercise. A new mother might need help in breaking the fast-food habit for herself and her children, replacing hamburgers and french fries with fruit and vegetables. We counsel sexually active women of all ages on how to use condoms and practice safe sex. And a tan never passes by without our commenting on how excess sun exposure increases the risk of skin cancer.

What we're doing, although we don't often say so directly, is teaching the women we see about primary cancer prevention. Primary prevention encompasses all the things people can do to affect their susceptibility to cancer and to protect themselves from cancer-causing agents.

As physicians, we also practice secondary cancer prevention. That means taking steps to detect and treat conditions that could lead to cancer. The tests we do and the observations we make as we practice secondary prevention sometimes border on cancer detection because in screening for precancerous conditions, we detect invasive cancers as well. For instance, a Pap smear to identify abnormal cells in the tissue covering the cervix may reveal cells that have become malignant. During a routine checkup we ask about our patients' family histories to determine their risk of inherited cancers.

PRIMARY PREVENTION

As you learned earlier, your genetic predisposition may lay the foundation for cells to go haywire and grow uncontrollably. But your diet, your exposure to the environment, and your habits—how you live your life day-to-day—play pivotal roles in the initiation and promotion phases of cancer development. Stopping cancer at those two points is what primary prevention is all about. Doing whatever you can to keep the cancer process from even starting is the most effective cancer-preventing step you can take. That's why we encourage our patients to scrutinize their lifestyles: Living a healthier life is the best defense against cancer.

You may assume you know all there is to know about a cancer prevention lifestyle, but adopting healthier habits can be a challenge. Understanding how and why a particular lifestyle factor or habit is linked to the cancer process often helps convince people to make healthy change. So here is an overview of what we know about primary prevention strategies. Later, when discussing the specific cancers, we'll give you more details, which those at high risk for that particular malignancy will find especially useful. And in part 3, we'll explain how you can make the lifestyle changes necessary to lower your personal cancer risk.

STOP SMOKING

At least a third of all cancer deaths in the United States result from cigarette smoking. According to the National Cancer Institute, tobacco use is the single most preventable cause of cancer death. Smoking is most often linked to lung cancer, but it can set the stage for cancer in any organ that tobacco or its some 4,000 known compounds make contact with. Even when tobacco smoke is not inhaled, its by-products make contact with some area of the body, like the lips or tongue.

Smokers are most likely to develop cancer of the lung; the larynx, or voice box; the oral cavity, including the lips, tongue, and mouth; the pharynx, or throat; and the esophagus, that portion of the digestive tract that extends from the mouth to the stomach. Smoking is also a contributing cause of cancer of the bladder, pancreas, cervix, kidney, stomach, liver, and colon and rectum, and of some types of leukemia.

No matter how you smoke your tobacco, there is a cancer risk. Cigar and pipe smokers are prime candidates for lung cancer, in addition to oral cancers. And tobacco use doesn't just mean smoking. Smokeless or "spit" tobacco, like chewing tobacco or snuff, also causes cancer. The National Collegiate Athletic Association has already banned spit tobacco, and the Little League has implemented an education program to discourage children from emulating the sports stars they see using it.

Researchers around the world are studying all aspects of this enormous problem, from basic biological research to epidemiologic studies analyzing the effects of smoking in large groups of people. Scientists are trying to determine precisely how tobacco contributes to cancer as well as how to keep people—particularly adolescents—from starting to smoke. They're also trying to learn the most effective way to help people quit once they've started.

Since 1950, when the first study showing a clear association between smoking and lung cancer was published, there has been no doubt that the surest way to reduce your risk of lung cancer was to not pick up a cigarette. But can quitting once you start give you a clean slate?

It's estimated that at least half of the nearly 172,000 cases of lung cancer diagnosed each year are in former smokers. It's not known how many of the 157,200 deaths from the disease each year would have been prevented if the smokers had quit a year or two after starting. But it is known that within 3 months of quitting, lung function improves up to 30 percent and risk of all types of lung cancer begins to decrease. Over the following months, lung function continues to improve. Your risk of cancer decreases the longer you have stopped smoking; this is particularly true among heavy smokers and among women.

If you've recently quit smoking, you'll soon notice that you feel less short of breath as the natural mechanisms that allow the lungs to cleanse themselves return to normal. Still, it will take a full 10 years for your risk of lung cancer to be about half that of your friends who are still smoking—depending, of course, on how many cigarettes you smoked and for how long. But no matter how old you are now or how long you've been smoking, keep in mind that it's never too late. A healthy man in his early sixties who quits smoking can reduce his risk of dying in the next 15 years by 10 percent.

You don't have to be a smoker to suffer its ill effects. Living with a smoker and working or socializing in an environment where there are people smoking puts you at risk, too. According to the Environmental Protection Agency, secondhand smoke causes about 3,000 deaths from lung cancer each year. And secondhand smoke from cigars is even worse. The American Cancer Society says that your chances of dying from lung cancer are 30 percent higher if you live with someone who smokes than if you lived in a smoke-free house. That statistic may help you convince others in your family to stop polluting the air you breathe.

Researchers are trying to learn if drugs such as retinoids and COX-2 inhibitors might reverse precancerous conditions in the lungs of heavy smokers and former ones. These studies are encouraging but have not yet come to a conclusion. For now, drugs are not substitutes for a healthy diet and a smoking cessation program.

ADOPT A HEALTHY DIET

A third of the 500,000 cancer deaths that occur in the United States each year are associated with poor diet and lack of exercise. According to report from the American Institute for Cancer Research and the World Cancer Research Fund, "Between 30 and 40 percent of all cases of cancer may be preventable by feasible and appropriate diets and by physical activity and maintenance of appropriate body weight. . . . On a global basis . . . this means that appropriate diet may prevent 3 million to 4 million cases of cancer every year. Diets containing substantial and varied amounts of vegetables and fruits will prevent 20 percent or more of all cases of cancer."

One of our patients, a breast cancer survivor, said to us that cancer research on diet always seemed to be a work in progress, and she's right. There are many very important dietary steps that a person can take to lower cancer risk—and we're going to fill you in on all of those—but as of this writing, there is not a single food, nutrient, or supplement about which we can say: Eat this and you won't get cancer. We can say, however, eat this way and you can reduce your risk. Cut this from your diet and you're less likely to get cancer. And in many cases we can offer you a plausible explanation. But research into what, how, and why diet causes or protects against cancer is indeed a work in progress, and the final conclusions have not been made.

FRUITS AND VEGETABLES. We do know that fruits and vegetables cut cancer risk, even though we aren't certain how they do it. What we've learned from studies thus far is that nutrient-rich, high-fiber, low-fat foods and a low-calorie diet reduce the risk of most cancers, including those in which another risk factor, such as tobacco, is involved.

Protein is essential for cell growth, but we don't know yet what role it plays in cancer prevention. Nor do we know why components of fruits and vegetables are protective. We know it's probably due to the vitamins, minerals, phytochemicals, fiber, or 2,000 plant pigments in fruits and vegetables, but we don't know with certainty how these things stop the cancer process.

Currently Americans eat barely two to three servings of fruits and vegetables a day. Five is the minimum to meet your nutritional needs, and we agree with the National Cancer Institute that nine should be your goal. However, we know this is really tough to do. Beginning on page 233, we'll show you how you can make achieving this goal easier.

GRAINS. Grains, too, seem to be protective, but as with fruits and vegetables, we don't know if the benefits are due to vitamins and minerals in whole grains, to the fiber, or to the protein. Perhaps it's all three, or perhaps certain grains are more protective than others.

MEAT. Meat is a mix of nutritional benefits and hazards. It provides high-quality protein and healthy vitamins and minerals. But in exchange,

many cuts also contain a lot of fat, particularly saturated fat and cholesterol. Some evidence indicates not only that these types of fat increase
the risk of heart disease but that saturated fat is associated with cancer.
Fish, in contrast, is a good source of protein and of omega-3 fatty acids,
which are good for your heart.

The way meat is cooked can pose a cancer risk, too. When protein is
cooked at a high temperature, carcinogenic compounds called heterocyclic amines are formed. The longer meat is cooked at high temperatures, the more of these substances are formed. According to the
Physicians Committee for Responsible Medicine, grilled chicken is an especially potent source of heterocyclic amines; it contains 15 times more
of these carcinogens than does roast beef or a hamburger.

Cooking meat at high temperatures, as with grilling or barbecuing,
also is a source of carcinogens known as polycyclic aromatic hydrocarbons
(PAHs). These are formed when bits of meat, fish, or chicken fall onto
the coals and the smoke then coats the surface of the grilling food. Some
people appear to be more susceptible than others to PAHs and HCAs.

CALORIES. One thing is certain: Consuming more calories than
you use leads to weight gain. And obesity—meaning having an excess of
body fat—increases a woman's risk of cancers of the breast (after
menopause) and gallbladder, as well as a man's risk of cancers of the
colon. Recently obesity has been implicated in cancers of the pancreas
and kidney.

In the spring of 2003, the largest-ever study to examine the correlation
between weight problems and cancer deaths revealed that being overweight or obese contributed to 14 percent of cancer deaths among men
and 20 percent among women. The death rates climbed among the heav-
iest cancer patients. The study also found higher death rates for cancers
not previously linked to obesity, including those of the esophagus, liver,
and colon and rectum, as well as non-Hodgkin's lymphoma and multiple
myeloma. The study authors concluded that as many as 90,000 cancer
deaths could be prevented if people would maintain a healthy body weight.

We don't know why obesity contributes to cancer, and we don't know
if losing weight, once you've put on too many pounds, lowers risk. What
we know is that maintaining a normal weight throughout life is associated

with a lower risk of cancer. Still, you've got nothing to lose by shedding those extra pounds. Along with preventing diabetes, stroke, and heart disease, losing excess weight can improve your overall health. It's especially important for young people to avoid gaining weight because once those pounds are there, they tend to accumulate through life.

KEEP MOVING

There is evidence that exercising for 45 minutes, 5 or more days a week, reduces the risk of some cancers, including breast and colorectal cancers. Regular moderate activity, like brisk walking, and vigorous exercise, such as jogging or taking an aerobic dance class, improve many body functions. Although improvements in heart and lung function are well-documented benefits of regular exercise, it's still not clear how physical activity affects the immune and endocrine systems, both of which might affect the cancer process. What we do know is that being sedentary increases the risk of certain cancers, and that being active helps to maintain a healthy body weight, which is an important step in cancer prevention.

One of the most important ways in which exercising cuts your risk of cancer is that it helps control your weight. Regardless of what you do— washing the car, running, climbing stairs—exercise burns calories, and if you manage to use more calories than you consume, you will shed the fat that's a depot for extra calories.

WATCH HOW MUCH YOU DRINK

The risks of all types of cancer increase in those who consume three or more alcoholic beverages a day. The risk increases 60 percent in heavy drinkers who average more than six drinks a day. And alcohol is associated with cancers of the mouth, pharynx, larynx, esophagus, liver, and breast.

When a smoker also drinks, he or she further increases the risk of cancers of the mouth, larynx, and esophagus. A landmark study that dramatically illustrates the impact of this deadly combination was done in the mid-1980s. Researchers found that if people consumed more than four drinks a day on average, their risk of oral and pharyngeal cancers increased ninefold. But if they were both heavy drinkers and heavy smokers, their risk jumped to 36 times that of those who didn't indulge in either habit!

The association between alcohol and cancer is so strong that the American Cancer Society says men should limit their intake to no more than two drinks a day, and women—because of their smaller size—to no more than one drink a day. Women at high risk for breast cancer may want to consider not drinking any alcohol. It's not known exactly how alcohol contributes to breast cancer, but among the current theories is that it increases estrogen levels. (See chapter 9.)

There's evidence that cutting back on alcohol consumption is protective. The American Institute for Cancer Research estimates that keeping alcohol intake within recommended limits would prevent up to 20 percent of cancers of the airway, upper digestive tract, colon and rectum, and breast.

PROTECT YOURSELF FROM THE SUN

In 2004, more than a million Americans were diagnosed with nonmelanoma skin cancers, which are either basal cell or squamous cell carcinomas. Although the nonmelanoma cancers are no longer life-threatening—99 percent are curable—the surgery to remove a skin cancer can be quite disfiguring, depending on the location and size of the lesion.

Melanoma, the most serious and life-threatening form of skin cancer, accounts for about 5 percent of skin cancers; about 55,000 new cases are expected to be diagnosed in 2004. All evidence points to excessive sun exposure as the primary risk factor for melanoma. The incidence increases in populations that live near the equator. However, because melanoma lesions can occur on parts of the body that are usually protected, the role of sunlight in this type of skin cancer is not clearly understood. A history of sunburn as a child and an intense blast of sun exposure seem to increase melanoma risk.

Ultraviolet radiation—especially the midlength UVB rays that cause sunburn—is a carcinogen. UVA rays are shorter and affect the immune system, which may ultimately contribute to cancer, too. Radiation from the sun damages the DNA in skin cells, but in most people those mutations are quickly repaired. One widely believed theory is that when these repairs are not made properly or completely, the cancer process begins. Also, with aging there is a decline in the cells' ability to repair themselves.

Tanning is a kind of injury, and it contributes to wrinkles, age spots, and thinning skin, as well as to skin cancer. And, despite what you read in the advertisements, a tan achieved with a tanning bed is not a "safe tan." In fact, tanning beds and tanning lamps may more than double the risk of skin cancer. People in one study who used either of these tanning devices were 2½ times more likely to develop squamous cell carcinoma and 1½ times more likely to have basal cell carcinoma than those who didn't use them. Tanning beds are also believed to increase the risk of melanoma.

Protecting yourself from UVB and UVA rays is the most important step you can take to prevent all types of skin cancer. Later in this book, you'll learn various ways to defend yourself from excessive sun exposure—wearing the appropriate sunblock being just one of them. There are certain treatments for the precancerous lesions that can become skin cancers that reduce your risk as well.

PRACTICE SAFE SEX

For nearly 100 years viruses have been suspected of causing cancer, but it's only since the 1980s and advances in molecular biology that scientists have been able to pinpoint specifically which types of viruses are responsible. As it turns out, many of these viruses are transmitted from one person to another through intimate contact. For instance, studies in the late 1980s showed that women who were infected with the sexually transmitted viruses that cause genital warts were 10 times more likely to develop cervical cancer than women who tested negative for the human papillomavirus (HPV).

Viruses cause infection by entering healthy cells, hijacking their DNA, and programming the cells to make infected cells instead of healthy ones. By finding fragments of DNA from the HPV virus in tumor cells from the cervix, researchers became convinced that HPV played a crucial role in cervical cancer. But HPV probably doesn't act alone. The theory is that other factors, such as smoking or other sexually transmitted infections, play a role in transforming healthy cells into malignant ones. Use of oral contraceptives and poor diet, for example, are believed to contribute to the persistence of HPV.

The herpes simplex virus type 2 (HSV-2), which causes infections in the mucous membranes, especially in the genital area, increase a woman's risk of cervical cancer two to four times. And it's quite widespread: The National Health and Nutrition Examination Survey reports that nearly one in five people in the United States carries HSV-2. Like HPV, infection with HSV-2 may never cause symptoms, and the person may be unaware he or she has it and unknowingly spread it to others.

Human immunodeficiency virus (HIV) infection is another viral infection linked to cancer, though the process is different from HSV-2 and HPV infection. HIV is transmitted in contaminated blood products or in bodily fluids, such as sperm, and it eventually may cause acquired immunodeficiency syndrome (AIDS). HIV destroys certain immune cells that normally defend the body, leaving the person susceptible to many infections and disorders, including cancer. One of the most common is Kaposi's sarcoma, a cancer that involves the lining of the blood vessels throughout the body.

Researchers have not yet pinned down what invades the body when immunity is suppressed and causes Kaposi's sarcoma, but they suspect an infectious agent is involved. That's because before AIDS, Kaposi's was a rare tumor. The number of people who developed it surged with the AIDS epidemic.

Although major advances are being made in developing vaccines against these and other viruses associated with cancer, your best defense right now is to protect yourself from infection. Later in this book, you'll learn specific safe sex practices that will prevent you from becoming infected and help you avoid transmitting to others viruses you might not even know you have.

WATCH THE X-RAYS

When radiation bombards a cell, its genetic material is damaged, and large amounts of radiation overwhelm the body's self-repair mechanisms. Just by virtue of living on earth, we're all chronically exposed to low levels of ionizing radiation in the atmosphere. The typical dose we get is about 1 to 2 gray a year. (A gray is an amount of radiation energy absorbed by the body.) For comparison, if a group of people were suddenly bombarded with 5 gray of whole-body radiation, about half of them would die within the month, according to the National Cancer Institute. The difference between that kind of sudden exposure and the background radiation in our environment is the time of exposure. Receiving 1 to 2 gray spread out over the year doesn't appear to pose a danger.

What you want to avoid is unnecessary sudden exposure, and except for a nuclear accident, that means avoiding unnecessary x-rays within a short period of time. A typical diagnostic x-ray delivers only 0.25 gray. Therefore, an annual mammogram poses little risk to women, even those at high risk for breast cancer.

Most physicians are well aware of the dangers of too much radiation, and if many diagnostic tests are needed, the doctors will consider the benefits of the tests versus the risks of the radiation exposure. Still, if you are seeing different doctors and dentists for various reasons, be sure that you let them know of any x-rays you have had within the past few years.

Medical radiation is the use of ionizing radiation to treat benign tumors and cancer. Since it typically involves larger doses of radiation than diagnostic x-rays, there is a risk that it can cause cancer. For instance, people who received radiation therapy in the 1950s to reduce an enlarged thymus gland are at increased risk of thyroid cancer and leukemia. At one time, enlarged tonsils and scalp ringworm were also treated with radiation. If you have ever had any kind of medical radiation treatment, let your physician know.

Today second cancers as a result of radiation therapy to treat cancer occur rarely, but the treatment does pose a risk. For example, teenagers who received chest radiation for Hodgkin's disease are at increased risk for breast cancer. A study of over 1,000 people of all ages treated with radiation for Hodgkin's disease found that they were at increased risk for leukemia, non-Hodgkin's lymphoma, melanoma, and cancers of the lung, breast, and stomach. Their risk was greatest if they received radiation therapy at a young age, and it declined with the age at which treatment began. Studies have shown that women who have had chest radiation are often unaware of their increased risk of breast cancer. It's important that they begin regular screening with mammography early.

Another source of radiation is radon in the earth and in building materials. It's estimated that 1 in 10 lung cancer deaths is related to this kind of exposure. Scientists first became aware of the dangers of radon, one of the substances created as uranium decays, when they noted the high incidence of lung cancer among uranium miners. Studies suggest that when radon is inhaled, it continues releasing radiation to the surrounding tissues, causing DNA damage and, eventually, cancer.

Now it's known that in certain areas where uranium is present in the soil, the levels of radon are higher than normal. The radon particles enter a building through the foundation and can reach toxic levels, particularly when windows and doors are tightly closed.

Homes can be easily and inexpensively tested, and if unhealthy levels of radon are detected, special pipes and fans can be used to adequately ventilate the house. For more information on radon testing, go the Environmental Protection Agency Web site at www.epa.gov.

We've learned so much about the dangers of radiation from studies of those who survived the atomic bomb explosions in Japan in World War II. In studies, women with tuberculosis who were monitored with frequent chest x-rays for 3 to 5 years had as high a rate of breast cancer as women who survived a single dose of radiation from the atomic bomb. This suggests that repeated small doses of radiation over an extended period of time may be as dangerous as a single large dose.

Mammograms are low-dose breast x-rays, and the benefits of detecting cancer early are thought to outweigh the small risk of developing cancer from annual mammograms, particularly for women over age 50 who are at increased risk for breast cancer.

KNOW YOUR JOB HAZARDS

There is a very long list of chemicals that are associated with cancer, and many of them are encountered in the workplace. In fact, one of the first causes of cancer to be identified was exposure to chemicals on the job. Today estimates vary widely, but carcinogens at work cause from 1 percent of cancers in one study to as many as 20 to 40 percent in another.

Because workers in certain industries come into contact more frequently with chemicals than does the average population, their illnesses, particularly cancer, are often a harbinger of what can affect all of us. Fortunately, once these carcinogens are identified, an effort can be made to control exposure to them.

One of the first known examples of an occupational cancer was the result of the epidemiologic study that made a connection between scrotum cancer and the soot that chimney sweeps were constantly exposed to. It wasn't until a century and half later that scientists learned why: Soot contains the carcinogen benzo[a]pyrene. From observations of miners in the mid-1800s, physicians learned that the miners were at high risk for lung cancer. But studies confirming the association between radon and lung cancer weren't done until nearly a century later, in the 1950s and 1960s.

Today, whenever people in a particular environment have a higher-than-normal incidence of a particular cancer, or a very unusual type of cancer appears to occur in workers in a particular industry, suspicions are aroused. At present there is no clearinghouse for this information, but studies of occupational hazards are continually being done. The International Agency for Research on Cancer (IARC), a branch of the World Health Organization, regularly publishes information on cancer risks from specific chemicals in various industries. The U.S. Department of Health and Human Services also publishes an annual report on carcinogens. You can access a complete list of known carcinogens on the IARC Web site at www.iarc.fr.

If you are frequently exposed to a chemical or process that you suspect may pose a danger, you might also check with your professional or occupational organization, if there is one.

This chapter is an overview of many of the changes you can make to lower your risk of cancer. But for specific recommendations of what we feel are the seven most important and basic cancer prevention steps that every person needs to begin doing today, see part 3.

CHAPTER 6

CHEMOPREVENTION

• • • • • • • • •

THE WORD *CHEMOPREVENTION* IS RELATIVELY NEW
to the vocabulary of cancer researchers, and is just beginning to filter out
of the laboratory to nonscientists. Most people are familiar with the word
chemotherapy, and know that it means using chemical agents to kill cancer
cells wherever they occur in the body. Chemoprevention involves using a
natural or synthetic substance—a nutrient or a drug—to keep cancer at
bay or to derail the disease process before cancer becomes invasive. In
other words, chemoprevention stops cancer from starting, or at least dis-
rupts the disease process before abnormal cells become full-fledged
cancer cells with a foothold in the body.

Chemoprevention began to emerge as a special field in cancer research in the late 1970s. Today it's one of the most exciting and
promising forms of primary cancer prevention available to us.

The basic principle behind chemoprevention is to change the way in
which cells behave. As you learned in chapter 1, the transformation of
healthy cells that reproduce at a normal rate into abnormal ones with the
capacity to grow wildly out of control happens in two phases: initiation
and promotion. Chemopreventives work by disrupting the two phases.
Those that shut down the initiation phase are known as blocking agents,
and those that interrupt the promotion phase, suppressing agents. Some
drugs and nutrients do both.

This overview is meant to acquaint you with the broad categories of
chemopreventives. In part 2, you will learn about the agents for specific

cancers, and whether they are currently available, in clinical trials, or still in development.

THE OPPORTUNITY FOR INTERVENTION

Chemopreventives perform their job in a variety of ways. Some stop the cellular transformation process by turning on or off a switch in a cell's genetic program. Some interfere with whatever is stimulating cellular reproduction—for example, by attaching to a hormone receptor on the surface of the cell so that the hormone responsible for cell growth and division can't find a place to attach. And some improve the body's ability to detoxify a harmful substance or to repair genetic damage caused by a virus.

According to chemoprevention pioneers, cancer is a fluid process, not an unchanging, static condition. The initiation phase may take place over hours or days, but the next phases—promotion and progression—may last as long as 20 years. Between the point where the cancer process starts and the point where the disease turns invasive is a huge window of opportunity for intervention.

We know that we have the capacity to prevent cancer because the reality is that most people do not get the disease during their lifetimes. The human body is equipped with mechanisms for defending against cancer, repairing genetic injury, and ridding itself of damaged cells before they grow out of control. Finding out how to optimize these mechanisms is the new frontier of cancer research.

In the early days, scientists studying cancer prevention concentrated their efforts on two approaches. One involved identifying the cause of a particular cancer and then avoiding it. For example, after research established a link between tobacco smoke and lung cancer, it quickly became clear that quitting smoking could lower cancer risk.

The second approach was to look for signs of a precursor or precancer—that is, a condition that could lead to cancer—or to identify very early stage, or preinvasive, cancer. The Papanicolaou smear, or Pap test, to detect abnormal lesions on the cervix became well-known in the mid-1950s, soon followed by mammography to detect cancerous changes in the breasts. Both screening tests remain important tools for secondary cancer prevention.

Ever since, scientists have continued to make advances in developing tests and identifying lifestyle changes that could lower cancer risk. By the 1970s, they were realizing that effective cancer prevention could include a third approach: actively targeting cancer-prone cells with chemopreventive substances.

PROMISE IN A PILL

Chemoprevention research was snowballing by the late 1970s and in full swing by the 1980s, when at least 70 trials of various chemopreventives were under way. In 1982, the National Cancer Institute established its Chemoprevention Branch to identify and test potential chemopreventive agents. Among the first to go under the microscope were the retinoids, the vitamin A derivatives discovered by pioneering chemoprevention researcher Michael B. Sporn, M.D. The retinoids had shown promise as a treatment for oral lesions that were likely to lead to cancer.

Today scientists are studying more than 400 compounds for possible chemopreventive actions. Of these, 40 are the subject of about 80 clinical trials. The largest-ever trial for chemopreventives, involving more than 30,000 men, began in 2001. It is evaluating the effectiveness of selenium and vitamin E in protecting against prostate cancer.

Thus far, the FDA has approved two drugs specifically for cancer prevention. One is tamoxifen, which can dramatically reduce the chances of breast cancer in women at high risk for the disease. The other is celecoxib for familial adenomatous polyposis, a condition that often leads to the onset of colorectal cancer at a young age. (We'll say more about both drugs later in the chapter.)

How many people ultimately will benefit from chemoprevention remains to be seen. Research is hinting at the potential for several categories of use. Until recently, many of the studies concentrated on people at highest risk for cancer—for example, those who have survived one bout with the disease and want to avoid a recurrence. Now a growing number of trials are bringing in people in other circumstances.

For example, a study might seek to identify substances that can reverse the development of a precancerous skin lesion. We already know that surgical removal of a lesion effectively prevents skin cancer. But research has shown that topical application of substances such as fluorouracil (5-FU) also can get rid of a lesion, thus reducing cancer risk.

Chemoprevention may have applications for those who inherited a genetic predisposition to cancer, such as women who carry the gene mutations for breast cancer. And it could be beneficial for those who are at risk for cancer because of environmental or lifestyle factors. One of the most exciting breakthroughs in chemoprevention is the development of a vaccine to protect against the sexually transmitted virus that infects about 20 percent of adults and is responsible for half of all cervical cancers.

Of course, chemoprevention can even help healthy people who are at normal risk for cancer. They, too, want to improve their odds of staying cancer-free for a lifetime.

THE CHEMOPREVENTIVES: A CLOSER LOOK

Right now, scientists are giving research priority to five classes of chemopreventives: retinoids; cyclooxygenase, or COX, inhibitors; nutrients such as calcium; hormone blockers; and vaccines. Some agents, like the hormone blocker tamoxifen, already are available but continue to undergo study. Some, like the hormone blocker finasteride, have performed well in trials but are not yet approved as chemopreventives. And some, like calcium, still need to be proven effective, though the research certainly looks promising.

Let's take a closer look at the five classes of chemopreventives, beginning with the retinoids. We'll explain how each class works, or is thought to work, and how they're faring in research.

RETINOIDS

Of all the chemopreventives, perhaps the most well-known and well-studied are the retinoids. You probably are familiar with beta-carotene, one of 500 carotenoids that give fruits and vegetables their yellow or orange color. Your body converts beta-carotene to vitamin A (also known as retinol) in the small intestine, then stores it in the liver until it's needed.

Although you can find some dietary sources of vitamin A—such as liver, fish-liver oil, and dairy products—most of the nutrient that circulates in your bloodstream started out as beta-carotene. So vitamin A, beta-carotene, and the thousand different synthetic retinoids all belong to the same nutritional family.

About 75 years ago, a Japanese scientist was the first to suggest that people who don't get enough vitamin A in their diets are more likely to develop cancer. Subsequently, researchers determined that when cells lining the throat, lungs, and cervix ran low on vitamin A, they changed in ways that could lead to cancer. Now we know that vitamin A plays a role in the development of healthy epithelial cells, such as those that line the mucous membranes—probably by regulating the function of certain genes in these cells. Because vitamin A supports differentiation, or normal cell growth, it is known as a differentiating agent. Interestingly, early experiments showed that giving vitamin A to animals deficient in the nutrient could restore healthy epithelial cells.

Despite scientific advances that helped solidify our understanding of the relationship between vitamin A and cancer, it wasn't until the 1970s that a large study confirmed that deaths from the disease were highest among people who had the lowest levels of beta-carotene in their blood. This study prompted many more scientists to investigate how beta-carotene and retinoids affect cancer risk.

Retinoids employ a number of strategies to prevent the transformation of healthy cells into malignant ones. They don't appear to make much of an impact during the initiation phase of the cancer process, when cells are first exposed to a cancer-causing substance. Rather, they take action later on, probably by interrupting the promotion phase.

Retinoids have demonstrated that they can reverse the cancer process in cells—at least in the laboratory. After successful testing in test tubes and animals, the next logical step was to try retinoids in humans. Large population studies already had suggested that vitamin A could protect against cancer. But in the 1990s, three important trials failed to confirm what scientists had seen in the laboratory. Supplements of beta-carotene, vitamin A, and vitamin E did not appear to have any protective effect. In fact, in two of the trials, those taking beta-carotene were *more* likely to develop lung cancer. This finding prompted researchers to question whether taking a nutrient or two is sufficient to interrupt the cancer process, and whether beta-carotene actually functions as an antioxidant.

In Finland, the Alpha-Tocopherol, Beta-Carotene Cancer Prevention Study Group—also known as the ATBC study—set out to determine if alpha-tocopherol (a form of vitamin E), beta-carotene, or both could reduce lung cancer in nearly 30,000 smokers. After 4 years, none of the supplement regimens showed a protective effect. Among those taking beta-carotene, the incidence of lung cancer increased by 18 percent, and overall deaths by 8 percent. By comparison, those taking alpha-tocopherol showed no major change in incidence of lung cancer or mortality. This study concluded that beta-carotene not only didn't help, it caused harm.

Similarly, the Carotene and Retinol Efficacy Trial—also known as the CARET study—compared the daily use of supplements (30 milligrams of beta-carotene and 25,000 IU of vitamin A) with a placebo in about 18,000 men and women at high risk for lung cancer. All of the participants were either smokers or former smokers. In addition, some of the men had worked with asbestos. The researchers stopped the trial 21 months early when they become convinced that the beta-carotene and vitamin A were doing more harm than good. By then the supplement group had tallied 28 percent more lung cancer diagnoses, and 17 percent more deaths, than the placebo group.

At the same time that the National Cancer Institute stopped the CARET study, it also released the results of the Physicians' Health Study, a landmark study involving more than 22,000 American physicians. It found no difference in the number of cancer deaths over the course of 12 years among people who took beta-carotene supplements and those who didn't. These results are another reminder that supplements are not yet proven as chemopreventives, and that cancer-fighting nutrients straight from whole fruits and vegetables remain a safer and healthier option for now. Good evidence suggests that eating fruits and vegetables may reduce your risk of several diseases, including certain cancers.

So what do we know about retinoids as chemopreventives? The animal studies certainly are promising, but with a few exceptions, the human research has been disappointing. Perhaps we still haven't discovered the one micronutrient that's responsible for the protective effects. Or perhaps we need to replicate and test a precise combination of micronutrients normally found in fruits and vegetables.

One drug that has shown promise, particularly for preventing ovarian cancer, is fenretinide, or 4-HPR. Researchers in Italy tested the drug, a retinoid product, in a group of women who were at high risk for ovarian cancer because they'd had breast cancer. Over the 5 years of the study, the incidence of ovarian cancer actually declined. More studies are under way to examine fenretinide's potential as a chemopreventive.

CYCLOOXYGENASE INHIBITORS

The enzyme cyclooxygenase plays an important role in the body's response to injury by prompting the production of prostaglandins, which in turn trigger an inflammatory reaction. The prostaglandins join with other chemicals to dilate blood vessels, increasing bloodflow and sending white blood cells to the site of the injury to destroy any invaders and remove cellular debris. As a result, the affected area becomes red, hot, swollen, and painful. But inflammation can affect the entire body, causing fever and loss of fluids from the blood.

Inflammation is a natural defense mechanism, but it can be overzealous at times. In arthritis, for instance, damage to the protective cartilage within a joint allows the bones that form the joint to rub together. The accompanying inflammation only aggravates the pain.

Cyclooxygenase appears to take two forms. One, called COX-1, is present in most normal tissues and primarily performs housekeeping functions within cells. In the cells that make up the stomach lining, for example, COX-1 prompts the flow of mucus to moisten the lining and to keep food moving through the digestive tract. The other form, COX-2, ordinarily is not present. Instead, it is produced in response to inflammation. It occurs in abundance in joints affected by arthritis.

For years people with arthritis have taken drugs that block cyclooxygenase, known as coxibs or COX inhibitors, to relieve their pain. Among these drugs are ordinary aspirin and nonsteroidal anti-inflammatory drugs (NSAIDs) such as diclofenac, ibuprofen, and naproxen. They counter inflammation by inhibiting both COX-1 and COX-2. Another drug, celecoxib, inhibits only COX-2.

In addition to inflamed areas, researchers have found cyclooxygenase in cancer cells from the head and neck, lung, pancreas, colon, and prostate, as well as in precancerous lesions and malignant tumors. It appears in benign tumors, too, though in much smaller amounts than in malignancies.

Whether and how COX-1 and COX-2 contribute to the development of cancer is the subject of ongoing study. From what we know so far, it may help stimulate angiogenesis—that is, the growth of new blood vessels to supply a tumor with nourishment. Somehow, too, it interferes with normal cell death, so damaged cells continue reproducing rapidly. Normal cell death, called apoptosis, is especially important in organs like the intestine, where healthy tissues constantly replace themselves. In addition, animal studies suggest that COX-2 may play a role in cases of breast cancer in which the patient carries the HER-2/neu gene.

The idea that cyclooxygenase might be a target for chemoprevention first surfaced in the 1990s. At the time, scientists already knew that the enzyme was abundant in cancer cells, and that drugs to inhibit the enzyme stopped cancer growth in animals. In experiments involving mice with intestinal polyps, the number of polyps declined once the gene that manufactures cyclooxygenase was disabled. Scientists also knew that the rates of colon polyps and colorectal cancer were lower among people with arthritis who had been taking COX inhibitors for years.

In a study of patients with familial adenomatous polyposis (FAP), a rare condition that eventually leads to colorectal cancer, taking celecoxib twice a day for 6 months reduced the number of new colon polyps by 28 percent. In addition, 23 of the 30 study participants experienced a decline in the number of existing polyps. This study convinced the FDA to approve celecoxib for people with FAP in December 1999. As a condition of approval, the manufacturer, Searle Monsanto, must continue studying the drug to monitor its safety and effectiveness and to provide further evidence that it will help people with FAP. Current research is focusing on whether starting therapy sooner rather than later will be even more effective in managing the condition. In another study, scientists are pitting celecoxib alone against celecoxib in combination with other drugs.

Researchers also are looking into whether celecoxib can prevent colorectal cancer in people with hereditary nonpolyposis colon cancer syndrome (HNPCC). An inherited condition, HNPCC raises the risk of colorectal cancer in both men and women, as well as the risk of endometrial cancer in women. About 75 percent of people with HNPCC develop cancer sometime in their lives.

Even people who don't have an inherited genetic predisposition to colon cancer might benefit from chemopreventive therapy with celecoxib. Clinical trials comparing the drug with a placebo are taking place at more than 50 centers across the United States and the United Kingdom. Studies of a related drug, rofecoxib, also are under way in the United States and Europe. And other coxibs—such as valdecoxib and etoricoxib—are in development.

Celecoxib's protective effects may extend well beyond colorectal cancer. Studies are investigating the drug's potential to heal precancerous lesions in the bladder and to treat and prevent actinic keratoses— the rough, scaly patches on the skin's surface that can turn into squamous cell skin cancer over time.

COX-2 inhibitors like celecoxib do have side effects. One report that analyzed the results of four separate studies raised concerns about the risk of heart problems and the possibility of the drugs' causing blood clots. In general, though, COX-2 inhibitors are better tolerated and safer than NSAIDs because they don't interfere with the housekeeping enzyme COX-1, which helps protects the stomach lining. Squelching

COX-1 can cause gastrointestinal side effects, including gastritis, ulcers, and bleeding.

Thus far, 30 of 32 studies examining the effects of NSAIDs on colon polyps and colorectal cancer have shown the drugs to be protective. But the Physicians' Health Study, which evaluated—among other things— whether taking 325 milligrams of aspirin every other day could lower the risk of death from heart disease, found that the drug did not lower the risk of colon polyps or colorectal cancer. What's more, daily doses of aspirin may interfere with blood clotting, while NSAIDs in general may cause kidney failure.

CALCIUM

Like many nutritional deficiencies with links to cancer, the idea that a low calcium intake might contribute to the disease came from studies involving large numbers of people. But the calcium–cancer connection is somewhat circuitous. It first surfaced when researchers noticed that a population's risk of cancer seemed to rise in proportion to its distance from the equator. Of course, the most obvious difference between the equator and places far from it is the amount of sun exposure.

Although we think of sun exposure as a cause of cancer, it also helps prevent the disease. The skin needs sun to manufacture vitamin D, which in turn is necessary for calcium absorption in the intestine. So people who live far from the equator may have a higher death rate from colorectal cancer because they don't make enough vitamin D and don't absorb enough calcium.

When researchers in Chicago set out to test this theory, they determined that men who consumed more vitamin D had a 50 percent lower incidence of colorectal cancer. The study also found that men whose calcium intakes exceeded 1,200 milligrams a day had a 75 percent lower incidence of colorectal cancer. The bottom line is, calcium by itself cannot prevent colorectal cancer; vitamin D is a critical component.

One possible explanation for calcium's protective effects is that it attaches to fat by-products, such as fatty acids and bile acids, and prevents them from irritating the intestinal walls. Normally the body responds to irritation by producing more cells to repair the injury. But as you learned in chapter 1, this increased cellular proliferation raises the possibility of cellular damage that could lead to cancer. It's possible, some researchers reason, to squelch the irritation with calcium.

Another explanation is that when calcium binds to fatty acids and free bile acids that are secreted by the liver, a substance is created that cannot pass through the intestinal wall into the bloodstream. Instead, it passes from the body. In effect, calcium escorts the offending acids from the body before they can be absorbed.

Animal studies support both of these theories. Meanwhile, four of five clinical trials involving humans determined that consuming a little more than the current Recommended Dietary Allowance of 1,000 to 1,200 milligrams of calcium a day inhibits the growth of cells lining the colon. This finding has led to even more studies to assess the mineral's role in cancer prevention.

Some scientists want to find out how calcium affects the return of tumors that already have undergone treatment. Since research on tumor recurrence can take years, they also are looking for biomarkers—early indicators of cell growth—that would reveal the mineral's impact much sooner. Other research groups hope to discover whether calcium therapy is most effective during a certain period of a tumor's development. Some recent studies suggest that the mineral may alter the chemistry of cells in many tissues of the body, ultimately affecting the cells' ability to develop completely.

Many experts predict that with further research, calcium and calcium-rich foods will prove to be important chemopreventives. What remains to be seen is whether calcium works best by itself or in combination with other substances.

HORMONE BLOCKERS

For decades, healthy women have been taking hormones to prevent pregnancy and to relieve the discomforts of menopause. We've seen how hormones can lower the risk of cancer in some organs and raise the risk in others. For example, the progesterone in oral contraceptives can help protect against ovarian cancer. But estrogen alone, without progesterone, can contribute to endometrial cancer. We still don't know for certain whether and how oral contraceptives influence breast cancer, though some experts believe that starting the Pill at a young age and taking it for a long time can elevate risk.

Hormones appear to have some role in directing cell division within the reproductive system. They also drive cell growth. How cells respond to hormones varies from one organ to the next. In women, for example, breast cells and endometrial cells behave differently in the presence of progesterone. Colon cells may react to hormonal stimulation as well.

In men, the prostate gland is under direct influence of male hormones, or androgens. One of these hormones, testosterone, converts to dihydrotestosterone (DHT) in the prostate at the direction of an enzyme called 5-alpha reductase. In June 2003, researchers called an early end to the Prostate Cancer Prevention Trial after they concluded that the drug finasteride—which inhibits the activity of 5-alpha reductase—could reduce the incidence of prostate cancer. (To learn more, see chapter 8.)

By far the most extensively researched hormone blocker, and the first drug to make the transition from cancer treatment to chemopreventive, is tamoxifen (Nolvadex). It's one of a new category of drugs called SERMs, short for selective estrogen receptor modulators. Another is raloxifene (Evista), which also is under investigation as a potential chemopreventive.

A SERM is a synthetic, or man-made, hormone that binds to estrogen receptors within the cells of certain tissues. As a result, molecules of the real hormone (estrogen) can't latch on to the receptors. That's why tamoxifen is known as an antiestrogen, even though it doesn't behave that way in all of the body's tissues.

Tamoxifen was one of several drugs synthesized in the 1960s. At the time, British researchers thought it might be useful to treat certain breast malignancies that were stimulated by the female hormone estrogen. Experiments involving laboratory rats had shown that tamoxifen caused cells to stop dividing and go into a resting state. Researchers suspected that the drug could destroy breast cancer tumors with none of the toxicity of traditional chemotherapy. Other antiestrogen drugs were in the pipeline, but tamoxifen appeared to have fewer toxic effects, and it worked in smaller doses.

The theory behind tamoxifen built on the observation, made decades earlier, that reducing a woman's estrogen supply by removing her ovaries or using radiation to destroy the ovaries could slow the progression of breast cancer, if not arrest it entirely. Interrupting estrogen flow was crucial, and tamoxifen could do that without surgery or radiation—as long as the tumor had estrogen receptors. Not all breast tumors do. (Incidentally, it now is standard practice for a pathologist to examine a breast tumor for estrogen receptors. If they are present, the cancer is said to be estrogen dependent, or estrogen receptor positive.)

Clinical trials using tamoxifen for women with advanced breast cancer, and then women with early-stage cancers, proved the theory right. In the 23 years since the drug's approval as a cancer treatment, its indications have expanded. Indeed, many breast cancer survivors are alive because of it.

Interestingly, the longer a woman takes tamoxifen, the greater the drug's benefits seem to be. Those who have been taking 20 to 40 milligrams a day for 5 years—the current maximum recommendation—experience a 50 percent reduction in their risk of cancer recurrence. Thus far, there's no proof that continuing tamoxifen therapy for more than 5 years is beneficial in cases where cancer has not spread to the lymph nodes.

What's more, tamoxifen appears to work equally well for women of all ages, whether they're pre- or postmenopausal. Women over age 70 who have taken the drug show a significant decline in the number of cancers that successfully make a comeback.

THE STUDY THAT STARTED IT ALL

It may seem like a small step from stopping recurrent breast cancers and second primary breast cancers to preventing the disease in healthy women. But proving that tamoxifen could do the job required a 4-year study involving 13,388 women. Known as the National Surgical Adjuvant Breast and Bowel Project (NSABP) Breast Cancer Prevention Trial, it launched in 1992 under the direction of physicians at 130 health centers across the country.

The primary objective of this study was "to determine whether tamoxifen administered for at least 5 years prevented invasive breast cancer in women at increased risk." The researchers also hoped to find out whether the drug could help prevent heart disease and bone fractures. And of course, they wanted to identify any potential side effects—particularly with regard to endometrial cancer and pulmonary embolism (blood clots that travel to the lungs), since tamoxifen could increase the risk of both.

The female volunteers, who agreed to take either 20 milligrams of tamoxifen or a placebo every day for 5 years, needed to meet certain criteria in order to enroll in the study. They qualified if they were age 60 or older, or if they were younger—between ages 35 and 59—but had personal histories of lobular carcinoma in situ, a noninvasive breast cancer. A younger woman also was eligible if her breast cancer risk equaled that of a 60-year-old, according to a computerized calculation called the Gail Model. This calculation considers the following factors.

- Whether any of a woman's first-degree female relatives—mother, sisters, or daughters—has a history of breast cancer
- Whether she has children, and if so, the age at which she first gave birth
- The number of biopsied breast lumps, especially if the woman has atypical hyperplasia, a condition involving a proliferation of abnormal but not malignant breast tissue
- The age at which she began menstruating

Volunteering for the study also required that women be in generally good health, with a life expectancy of at least 10 years. They could not be on estrogen replacement therapy; if they were of childbearing age, they could not be pregnant or planning to become pregnant or be using oral contraceptives. They also underwent tests to confirm that they did not have any preexisting liver, kidney, or vein problems. If a woman satisfied all these criteria, and if a recent mammography and breast examination by a physician confirmed that she did not have breast cancer, she became a candidate for the study.

In 1997—7 years after the National Cancer Institute invited scientists to take a closer look at the possibility of reducing breast cancer risk with tamoxifen, and 6 years after the FDA gave its blessing to NSABP to conduct a clinical trail—the recruiting phase was complete. Each of the more than 13,000 participants was randomly assigned to one of two groups. All the women took a small white pill every day—but the pill for one group contained 20 milligrams of tamoxifen, while the pill for the other was a placebo. To avoid bias among the physicians who would periodically examine the women and collect data, no one knew who was taking which pill, unless necessitated by a life-threatening event.

WHAT NSABP FOUND

The study ended on March 24, 1998, with the first analysis of the data released shortly thereafter. By then 13,175 women had taken either tamoxifen or a placebo for an average of 47.7 months.

The initial results were very impressive. The incidence of noninvasive or invasive breast cancer was twice as high in the placebo group (244 cases) as in the tamoxifen group (124 cases). With regard to invasive breast cancer in particular, the incidence dropped from 175 cases in the placebo group to 89 in the tamoxifen group. Of the nine women who died of breast cancer during the course of the study, six had been taking the placebo, and three tamoxifen.

The reduction in breast cancer risk was especially significant among those with atypical hyperplasia, a benign condition that nevertheless is a breast cancer risk factor. Of the 614 women with the condition who took the placebo, 23 developed invasive breast cancer. By comparison, only 3 cancers occurred among the 579 women in the tamofixen group with atypical hyperplasia. Furthermore, the malignancies in the tamoxifen takers were less likely to have spread to the lymph nodes under the arm.

To the researchers involved in the clinical trial, these results clearly demonstrated that tamoxifen worked. By proving that a drug could lower breast cancer risk in those who took it, this landmark study ushered in the chemoprevention era.

Along with the positive results for breast cancer prevention, the NSABP trial generated data on side effects and complications that were similar to those from earlier studies of tamoxifen. Specifically, women taking the drug were 2.53 times more likely to develop invasive endometrial cancer than those taking a placebo. Of all the cases—36 in the tamoxifen group, 15 in the placebo group—27 occurred in women age 50 or older. The increased risk of endometrial cancer appears to concentrate in this older demographic.

From earlier studies, the researchers knew that tamoxifen could cause a slight increase in bone density in women who've gone through menopause. After 5 years of treatment, they're less likely to break a bone because of osteoporosis. The NSABP trial produced similar findings.

With regard to blood clots that could lead to stroke or pulmonary embolism, the women on tamoxifen were more likely to develop deep-vein blood clots than those on the placebo—35 cases versus 22. Likewise, the incidence of stroke was higher in the tamoxifen group (38 cases) than in the placebo group (24 cases). Pulmonary embolism, though rare, occurred in three times as many women on tamoxifen (18) as on the placebo (6). As with endometrial cancer, the risk of pulmonary embolism

How Tamoxifen Raises Endometrial Cancer Risk

Scientists once thought that when estrogen molecules attached to their receptors—and every cell contains thousands of them—it immediately prompted the transmission of messages to specific genes within the cell, triggering the division process. So by taking the place of estrogen in the receptor, tamoxifen could block the cascade of events leading to cell division.

Recently, though, research has shown that the antiestrogen effect is not as simple as flipping a genetic on-off switch. In some tissues, such as those in the endometrium, tamoxifen doesn't act like an antiestrogen at all. In fact, it turns on cell growth by mimicking the effects of estrogen. For this reason, women taking tamoxifen to prevent breast cancer require close monitoring for endometrial cancer.

appeared to be highest in women ages 50 and older. Regardless, physicians routinely inform their patients who take tamoxifen of the signs and symptoms of these conditions.

Since tamoxifen had produced menopauselike discomforts in previous studies, the researchers felt it was important to evaluate how the drug might affect quality of life. If it created too many disruptions and inconvenient side effects, women wouldn't take it consistently. The researchers wanted to know whether the study participants experienced symptoms such as hot flashes, irregular periods, fluid retention, and depression—and, if they did, whether these side effects significantly interfered with their lifestyles.

According to the participants' reports, the only difference between the two groups involved hot flashes and vaginal discharge. Among those taking tamoxifen, 45.7 percent said they had experienced "bothersome" hot flashes. This figure dropped to 28.7 percent among those taking the placebo. Similarly, 29 percent of those in the tamoxifen group complained of vaginal discharge, compared with 13 percent in the placebo group.

Physicians who recommend tamoxifen to female patients to reduce their breast cancer risk will carefully describe the possible side effects and contraindications of chemopreventive therapy, as well as its potential benefits. For example, even if a woman is of childbearing age, she may experience menopauselike discomforts, most commonly hot flashes. They can occur in women past menopause, too. In fact, according to a report in the *New England Journal of Medicine,* hot flashes are the most common adverse effect: "At least 50 percent of women treated with tamoxifen report hot flashes, but so do 20 to 40 percent of women given a placebo." Vaginal discharge also is common, occurring in about one-third of women who take the drug.

MORE ANSWERS, MORE QUESTIONS

As a result of the NSABP trial, a panel of advisors to the FDA unanimously recommended that the agency approve the use of tamoxifen to reduce the chances of breast cancer in women at high risk for the disease. While

scientists are convinced that tamoxifen and other SERMs may help reduce breast cancer risk, they still don't know exactly how the drugs work.
In the case of tamoxifen, for example, does it actually keep the cancer
process from starting, or does it somehow reverse the process after it already is under way? Or does it do both?

Another unanswered question pertains to the duration of tamoxifen
therapy. Is 5 years long enough, or would extending the treatment period
also extend the benefits? Follow-up research suggests that the protective
effects of tamoxifen last longer than the 5 years of treatment.

And finally, do the benefits of the drug outweigh the risks, especially
with regard to endometrial cancer and blood clots? For women under
age 50, the answer is yes. Those age 50 and older need to consider the
benefits and risks on an individual basis.

These days, researchers are concentrating their investigative efforts
on other SERMs that may produce benefits similar to tamoxifen's, but
with fewer side effects and less risk of other health problems. In 1999, the
Study of Tamoxifen and Raloxifene (STAR)—one of the largest-ever
breast cancer prevention trials—began recruiting women who are at increased risk for breast cancer at more than 500 centers in the United
States, Puerto Rico, and Canada. The enrollment criteria are the same as
for the NSABP trial, except that STAR is limited to postmenopausal
women. (A separate study is examining whether raloxifene is safe for pre-
menopausal women.)

Research involving raloxifene already has shown that women who
take the drug to treat and prevent osteoporosis are less likely to develop
breast cancer than women taking a placebo. So researchers designed the
5-year STAR study, currently under way, to compare the protective effects
of raloxifene and tamoxifen in postmenopausal women and to determine
if raloxifene is safe for long-term use.

Beyond SERMS, a new class of drugs called aromatase inhibitors—
which researchers are evaluating as treatments for breast cancer—one
day may prove to be effective preventives as well. As their name suggests,
aromatase inhibitors work by limiting the activity of aromatase, an enzyme that is necessary to produce estrogen. By disrupting production of

the hormone, these drugs discourage the growth of breast tumors that are sensitive to it.

In October 2003, the results of an international trial involving more than 5,000 women revealed that for postmenopausal women with breast cancer who had been on tamoxifen for five years, taking an aromatase inhibitor called letrozole (Femara) for an additional five years could reduce cancer recurrence by 43 percent. Several other trials evaluating various aromatase inhibitors currently are underway.

VACCINES

For years scientists have been experimenting with vaccines as treatments for several types of cancer. But in 2002 a research team published the first-ever study to show that a vaccine actually could prevent infection with a virus linked to cancer. The virus, a sexually transmitted human papillomavirus called HPV-16, is a known cause of cervical cancer. In fact, experts suspect that most of the 450,000 cases of cervical cancer that occur around the world each year result from infection with one of five types of HPV. Of these, HPV-16 has the strongest connection to cancer.

For the study, more than 2,000 young women who were free of HPV-16 infection received three injections of either HPV-16 vaccine or a placebo over a 6-month period. They were screened for the virus 1 month after the third injection and every 6 months thereafter. Seventeen months after the final injection, none of the women in the vaccine group had developed HPV-16 infection. By comparison, 49 in the placebo group had become infected. What's more, nine of these women showed abnormal growths on the cervix related to HPV-16 infection.

The HPV-16 vaccine is a real breakthrough. In combination with regular cervical cancer screening, it actually could put an end to cervical cancer, which is responsible for 2 percent of all cancer deaths among American women each year and is the second leading cause of cancer-related deaths among women throughout the world. Experts believe that if before women became sexually active they were vaccinated against the five types of HPV implicated in cervical cancer, their cancer risk would drop by 85 percent. Research is under way to develop vaccines that target three other types of HPV—HPV-18, HPV-6, and HPV-11.

THE WAVE
OF THE FUTURE

Chemoprevention is the next frontier in cancer research. True, some of the studies that we've presented here—and others that you will be hearing about in the future—produced mixed or even negative results. But we've seen so many positive results and breakthrough developments—tamoxifen for breast cancer, finasteride for prostate cancer, and the HPV-16 vaccine for cervical cancer—that we and many of the world's leading cancer experts believe in the promise of chemopreventive approaches.

Today, about 3 decades after cancer researchers first broached the idea of chemoprevention, this area of research is growing exponentially, particularly with regard to the five classes of chemopreventives presented in this chapter. Priorities have been set, study protocols designed, opportunities identified, and strategies for using them developed. All of these exciting advances are helping to attract a growing number of scientists to the chemoprevention field.

As we've seen, it takes large clinical trials conducted over many years to determine whether a specific substance can reduce cancer risk. But the promise of chemoprevention is greater than ever before.

· · · · · · · · **·** · ·

PART II

SELF-CARE
TO OUTSMART

9 COMMON

CANCERS

● ● ● ● ● ● ● ● ●

*D*uring the late 1990s, several medical breakthroughs forever changed the way we look at cancer. The most significant of these occurred at an annual meeting of cancer experts from around the world, with the announcement of the results of a landmark study that identified a completely new approach to obliterating cancer. Unlike chemotherapy, which uses drugs to destroy abnormal cells, this novel therapy—called chemoprevention—involved taking a drug to prevent cells from becoming abnormal in the first place.

Researchers had produced solid evidence that the drug tamoxifen (Nolvadex) actually could prevent breast cancer by stopping the female hormone estrogen from stimulating cancer cells. Among 13,000 women who took part in the National Surgical Adjuvant Breast and Bowel Project (NSABP) Breast Cancer Prevention Trial, tamoxifen produced an almost 50 percent reduction in the incidence of breast cancer among those at high risk for the disease.

That tamoxifen could dramatically lower the chances of breast cancer in women especially vulnerable to it was nothing short of a revelation. For the first time, physicians could offer patients the opportunity to control their risk for the disease. It was the dawn of a new era in the battle against cancer. As Harmon J. Eyre, M.D., medical director of the American Cancer Society, told a reporter, "This is the first absolutely convincing proof that the concept of chemoprevention works. . . . These studies have proven that you can prevent breast cancer by taking a pill. It's not just a hypothesis anymore." Today tamoxifen is the only drug with FDA approval for breast cancer risk reduction.

The results of the 5-year NSABP study, which had the support of the National Cancer Institute, prompted a great deal of excitement among oncologists and the news media. Several other studies also wrapping up the same year supported the notion that we can thwart the cancer process. For example, at Fox Chase Cancer Center in Philadelphia, research trials involving smokers indicated that a compound called oltipraz improved cell abnormalities associated with cancer in the lining of the lungs. And in another study with the backing of the National Cancer Institute, a research team from the Cleveland Clinic and Ohio State University found that a compound called suldindac reversed some precancerous intestinal conditions.

Preliminary reports from other trials added to excitement. At Fox Chase Cancer Center, a synthetic compound called finasteride (Proscar) appeared to prevent prostate cancer.

The study of these chemopreventive agents, as well as new ones, continues today. Entire textbooks, journals, and international meetings exist for the primary purpose of sharing scientific data about chemoprevention. According to the International Agency for Research on Cancer, "Chemoprevention has the potential to be a major component of cancer control. . . . This research has provided an opportunity to challenge cancer on an entirely new front and to bring us closer to the ultimate goal of worldwide cancer control."

WHAT WE KNOW ABOUT NUTRIENTS

In addition to drugs, researchers at medical centers throughout the world are involved in studies to see how specific components of food, and diet in general, influence cancer growth. But people are so eager to learn what they can do to stop cancer that sometimes the news gets a bit ahead of the reality. Nearly every day you can read an article or hear a sound byte about how a study has found that a certain vitamin, mineral, or plant compound (phytochemical) can prevent cancer. The truth is, we have very little proof of the protective properties of specific nutrients.

One small study is only one brick in the building of evidence to support good nutrition as a weapon against cancer. We need more bricks to lay a solid foundation for making dietary recommendations. That said, we are seeing more and more studies involving large groups of people in which dietary patterns—what and how people eat—can affect cancer risk.

For instance, although we don't know how dietary fat contributes to cancer, we do know that people who consume a lot of fat are more likely to develop certain cancers, such as breast cancer and colorectal cancer. We also know that people who consume a specific amount of fiber are less likely to develop colorectal cancer. We have theories about why fiber helps, but right now we can't say that you can avoid colorectal cancer by taking a fiber supplement.

You can lower your risk of cancer in general by making sure to include adequate amounts of fruits and vegetables in your diet. Even how you prepare your food can have an impact: Research has linked the by-products of charcoal grilling to stomach and colorectal cancers.

Outsmarting Our Genes

Renowned British epidemiologist Sir Richard Peto once wrote, "Cancer arises from three things: nature, nurture, and luck." When he made that observation more than 20 years ago, healthy nurturing—which for many involves a change in lifestyle—was about the only hope for cancer prevention. Now that scientists have unlocked some of the mysteries of genetics, including mapping the human genome, we're more optimistic. We're learning that we can get an edge on nature, too.

With genetic testing, for instance, we can identify inherited genetic mistakes that may raise the risks for certain cancers. We also have tools to look for certain cancer indicators, or biomarkers, in their earliest stages. Then, by taking immediate action to treat these precancers, we can stop the disease before it starts. At the very least, we can use routine screening tests to detect cancer early on, when the chances for cure are best. More of these tests are in the pipeline.

In the laboratory, scientists are learning more about the genetic mistakes that cause healthy cells to go awry, and about nutrients and drugs that can correct these mistakes and improve the body's natural ability to fight them. With each clinical trial and each discovery of a new preventive measure, the chances of avoiding a malignancy rise. As a result, the role of luck in determining whether a person develops cancer is becoming ever smaller.

More Breakthroughs to Come

The evidence that we can intervene in the cancer process is so strong that the National Cancer Institute has established two divisions devoted to cancer prevention. More than 400 compounds—including vitamins, minerals, hormones, and drugs—are under investigation as possible preventives, with more than 40 clinical trials currently ongoing. In the chapters that follow, we'll identify the key trials that may turn up new preventive measures for each particular cancer.

We believe that everyone can take steps to lower their cancer risk, including but not limited to treatment with chemopreventive drugs. We believe that with the appropriate tools, we can detect and treat precancers before they mushroom into full-blown cancer. And we believe that we can stop recurrences in those who already have done battle with the disease.

The optimal time to begin fighting cancer is when you are strong and vital. Because most cancers take years to develop, and most people who die from the disease are over age 40, your best bet is to take preventive action *now*, no matter what your age.

Deciding how far to go in your efforts to prevent cancer is a highly personal matter. The steps will vary with individual risk. Consider a woman whose mother and sister have breast cancer. Rather than take tamoxifen, she may opt for surgical removal of her breasts to protect against the disease, especially if testing reveals that she carries the genetic mutation for it.

Although about 90 percent of us don't have the sort of family history that would put us at highest risk for cancer, we still have some risk. After all, we're getting older, and age is among the most influential risk factors for cancer. We may not be able to turn back the clock. But we can do a great deal to improve our chances of living a long, cancer-free life.

The idea of being able to prevent cancer is very similar to taking steps to avoid heart disease, our nation's number one killer. In fact, the use of cholesterol-lowering drugs to intervene against heart disease convinced many scientists that the same approach—chemoprevention—might work to combat cancer. If people at risk for heart disease modify their diets, get more exercise, and take medication to lower their cholesterol and perhaps their blood pressure, why not use diet, exercise, and chemoprevention to lower cancer risk, too?

CHAPTER 7

MELANOMA

AND

OTHER

SKIN CANCERS

• • • • • • • • • • • • • •

SKIN CANCERS ARE THE MOST COMMON of all cancers, affecting more than a million people a year. By some estimates, 40 to 50 percent of us will develop a skin cancer sometime in our lives.

In general, skin cancers fall into two broad categories: melanomas and nonmelanomas. Melanomas originate in the pigment-producing cells known as melanocytes, while nonmelanomas arise from the cells that comprise the uppermost layer of skin, called the epidermis. The latter category includes basal cell cancers, which begin in cells at the bottom of the epidermis, and squamous cell cancers, which begin within the epidermis itself. (Another kind of skin cancer, Kaposi's sarcoma, primarily affects people with AIDS.)

Both basal and squamous cell cancers are quite common, affecting about a million people a year. The good news about them is that they rarely spread. But they must be removed, and depending on where they're located and how large they are, the surgery can be disfiguring.

Melanoma, in contrast, can be quite serious because it can spread quickly. The number of deaths from this form of skin cancer has climbed by about 44 percent since 1973, though fortunately its mortality rate has remained stable over the past decade. Still, according to the American Academy of Dermatology, one person dies from melanoma every hour.

In 2004, as many as 55,100 Americans could develop melanoma, making it the fifth most common cancer among men and the seventh most common among women. Experts attribute the prevalence of the disease to a combination of excessive unprotected sun exposure and a diminishing ozone layer that allows more of the sun's rays to reach the earth.

Not all melanomas are alike. For example, some spread across the skin before invading deeper tissue. And one type, nodular melanoma, usually already has become invasive by the time it is diagnosed.

Although melanomas account for just 10 percent of all skin cancers, they are responsible for 75 percent of all skin cancer deaths. This is because they are much more likely than basal cell or squamous cell carcinomas to spread to other parts of the body. In light of the seriousness of melanomas, we've chosen to focus on them here. But much of the information on risk, cause, and prevention applies to all kinds of skin cancer, unless specifically noted otherwise.

ARE YOU AT RISK?

1. ARE YOU CAUCASIAN? Melanoma can affect anyone, regardless of skin color. But Caucasians are at highest risk. Compared with African-Americans, for example, Caucasians are 20 times more likely to develop melanoma.

2. DO YOU HAVE FAIR SKIN? A person with fair skin is about four times more likely to develop skin cancer than a person with olive skin. People with dark skin are at low risk, though they still can get melanoma—usually on their palms or soles, or under their nails.

3. IS YOUR HAIR NATURALLY RED OR BLOND? If so, you're two to four times more likely to develop melanoma than someone with hair of another color.

4. HAS ANY FIRST-DEGREE RELATIVE—A PARENT, SIB-LING, OR CHILD—BEEN TREATED FOR MELANOMA? While only 5 to 10 percent of those diagnosed with melanoma report a family history of the disease, having a first-degree relative with the disease more than doubles your risk.

5. HAVE YOU EVER HAD A MELANOMA? If you already have been treated for one, you stand a 5 percent chance of developing another one.

6. DO YOU HAVE MANY MOLES, ESPECIALLY UN-USUAL ONES? About half of melanomas arise from moles—or nevi, as doctors call them. Particularly risky are those that are large or varied in color, or that have irregular borders. These are known as atypical, or dysplastic, nevi, and they tend to appear on a person's chest, back, abdomen, and legs.

7. WERE YOU BORN WITH ANY MOLES? Between 3 and 8 percent of melanomas occur in congenital moles. Although even a small congenital mole can develop into melanoma, the risk associated with larger moles—what are known as giant congenital nevi—is especially high. About 15 percent of these moles develop into melanomas.

8. DO YOU LIVE IN THE SOUTHERN UNITED STATES OR THE MIDWEST? Sunlight is more intense in the south than in the north. Recently, though, researchers traced the highest sunburn rates to the Midwest. In a 1999 survey, respondents from Indiana, Wisconsin, Utah, and Wyoming—as well as Washington, D.C.—reported more sunburns than any other part in the country. Why Midwesterners are more sunburn-prone remains to be seen, though some experts suggest that people generally don't wear sunscreen every day—only during the spring and summer, and then only when they're outdoors for extended periods of time.

9. DID YOU GET A LOT OF SUN EXPOSURE AS A CHILD OR A TEENAGER? Americans tend to get 80 percent of their

The Skin

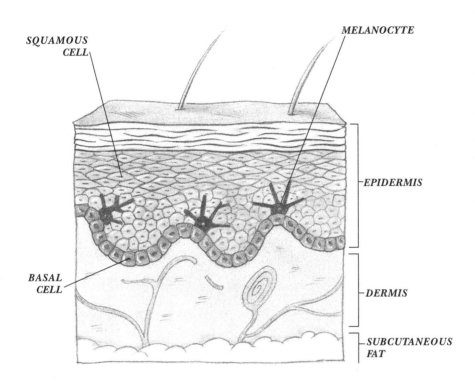

SQUAMOUS CELL

MELANOCYTE

EPIDERMIS

BASAL CELL

DERMIS

SUBCUTANEOUS FAT

SKIN CANCERS GET THEIR NAMES FROM THE CELLS IN WHICH THEY ORIGINATE. MELANOMAS BEGIN IN THE PIGMENT-PRODUCING MELANOCYTES, WHILE NON-MELANOMA SKIN CANCERS ARISE FROM SQUAMOUS OR BASAL CELLS.

sun exposure, and sun damage, before age 18. According to recent studies, even one severe or extensive sunburn after age 20 doubles melanoma risk. So, too, does getting five or more sunburns at any time in life.

10. DO YOU FREQUENTLY USE A SUN LAMP OR TANNING BED, OR VISIT TANNING SALONS? UV radiation from any source increases your melanoma risk. Advertisements often tout tanning beds as not producing UVB rays, which are responsible for much of the damage to the upper layer of skin. In fact, most beds emit small amounts of both UVB and UVA rays.

11. DO YOU WORK OUTDOORS OR SPEND A LOT OF TIME IN THE SUN FOR ANY REASON? One type of melanoma, lentigo maligna melanoma, commonly occurs with accumulated sun exposure. It accounts for about 5 percent of all melanomas.

12. ARE YOU USING A DRUG OR ANOTHER TREATMENT THAT WOULD SUPPRESS YOUR IMMUNE SYSTEM? Some experts believe that weakened immunity might allow some cancer cells to escape the body's own natural defenses.

13. DO YOU HAVE AN IMMUNODEFICIENCY DISEASE, SUCH AS AIDS OR LYMPHOMA? Your melanoma risk is four to five times higher in the presence of an immunodeficiency disease.

14. DO YOU HAVE XERODERMA PIGMENTOSUM? This rare genetic disease can dramatically increase melanoma risk.

CAUSES

Like most cancers, melanoma doesn't come from a single cause. Rather, it's the end result of an interaction between several factors, some of which scientists haven't even identified yet. Because the risk is so high in people who get a lot of ultraviolet radiation, excessive sun exposure likely plays a major role. In fact, in 2003 the federal government officially declared ultraviolet radiation a carcinogen.

We know that UVA rays do damage to the DNA of melanocytes, and that this damage continually undergoes repair. In cases of melanoma, some researchers theorize, people may carry a genetic defect that robs them of the necessary enzyme to engineer cellular repair. As a result, cells aren't fixed properly, if they're fixed at all.

In addition, because sun exposure suppresses the immune system, cells with damaged DNA aren't destroyed, as they normally would be. Instead, they survive and multiply.

UVB, the sun's burning rays, are thought to be responsible for much of the damage to the DNA in cells in the upper layer of the skin. But researchers believe that UVA rays, which penetrate deeper than UVB rays, can suppress the entire immune system and therefore affect the entire body. Even low doses of ultraviolet radiation can knock out Langerhans cells, specialized immune cells that are vital to the skin's defenses. Suppressed immunity also may explain why melanomas sometimes show up on areas of the body that are not directly exposed to sunlight.

Often melanomas occur in moles, which are clusters of melanocytes. Moles tend to appear by the time a person turns 20. Any changes in a mole—in terms of size, color, or sensation, like itching—are signs that it has become malignant.

While most people who develop melanoma have no family history of the disease, about 10 percent can identify at least one first-degree relative—a parent, sibling, or child—who has it. This isn't so surprising when you consider that family members may live in the same environment, eat the same diet, and follow the same lifestyle—all of which contribute to their cancer risk.

Some people, probably fewer than 1 or 2 percent, carry genetic mutations that predispose them to melanoma. Among those with family histories of the disease, it isn't unusual for several melanomas to appear at once, or for the cancer to develop at an early age.

In cases of hereditary melanoma, scientists have identified mutations in two genes that produce a growth-controlling protein called p16. One of the genes, CDKN2A, occurs in about 20 to 40 percent of families in which three or more first-degree relatives have melanoma.

As with other hereditary cancers, carrying the genetic mutation for melanoma doesn't mean that you automatically get the disease. It may depend on several other factors, such as whether you've gotten a lot of sun exposure or if you've inherited other genes that may affect your risk. According to one study, a person who inherits the so-called p16 gene has a 65 percent chance of developing melanoma before age 80.

Because the number of people with a genetic predisposition to melanoma is quite small, cancer experts continue to debate whether genetic testing in these cases is useful. The Melanoma Genetics Consortium suggests that those at high risk for melanoma who are considering genetic testing enroll in a clinical trial. It's the only way to find out for certain whether the testing improves early detection and saves lives. People with strong family histories of melanoma should have more frequent skin checkups, regardless of whether they choose to undergo genetic testing. So the question is, could this testing improve their watchfulness, and that of their doctors?

SCREENING

Both the Skin Cancer Foundation and the American Cancer Society recommend that you examine your own skin once a month for suspicious moles or other lesions. We recommend doing this self-exam while completely nude in front of a full-length mirror, using a hand mirror to inspect areas that are difficult to see directly.

Pay particular attention for new moles as well as for moles that look different or seem to be growing. A helpful aid for remembering the sorts of changes that require further examination by your physician is the abbreviation ABCD:

- A for asymmetry
- B for border irregularity
- C for color variation
- D for diameter—usually larger than ¼ inch, or about the size of a pencil eraser

The authors of a 1998 study suggested expanding this abbreviation to include E, for enlargement. You may be familiar with other self-exam aids as well. For example, one recommends watching for the three Cs: color, contour, and change.

The purpose of these tools is to help spot suspicious changes in moles. Inspect each mole for one half that doesn't match the other; ragged, notched, or blurred borders; varying shades of tan, brown, or black, or a mottled appearance with traces of red, white, and blue; or large or increasing size. If you notice anything unusual, see your doctor immediately.

If you have a sore that doesn't heal or that crusts, bleeds, or turns red, it may be a nonmelanoma skin cancer. It also should be checked out by your doctor.

How to Spot Melanoma

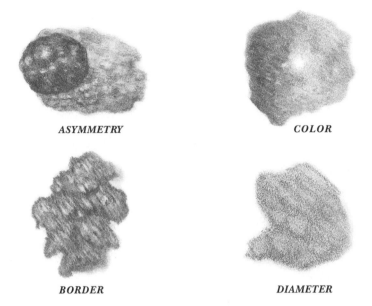

ASYMMETRY   COLOR

BORDER   DIAMETER

WHEN PERFORMING YOUR SKIN SELF-EXAM, REMEMBER ABCD: ASYMMETRY;
BORDER IRREGULARITY; COLOR VARIATION; AND DIAMETER LARGER THAN ¼ INCH.
A MOLE WITH ANY OF THESE CHARACTERISTICS REQUIRES FURTHER INSPECTION
BY YOUR DOCTOR. THEY MAY INDICATE THE PRESENCE OF MELANOMA.

To augment the monthly skin self-exam, the American Cancer Society recommends that a doctor inspect your skin as part of a regular
cancer-related checkup. The guideline for these checkups is every 3
years for people between ages 20 and 40, and every year for those age 40
or older.

If you're at high risk for melanoma, the American College of Preventive Medicine (ACPM) recommends a periodic total skin exam by a physician. According to the ACPM, "high risk" means that you have a family or
personal history of skin cancer, that you're exposed to sunlight on your
job or in your leisure time, or that you have dysplastic or congenital nevi.
The ACPM does not specify how frequent "periodic" might be.

In families where two or more people develop melanoma, the National Cancer Institute (NCI) urges any first-degree relatives—parents, siblings, and children older than age 10—to be examined for dysplastic nevi or any sign of melanoma. Based on this initial screening, their doctors can decide how often to follow up. For example, a doctor may recommend a total skin exam every 6 months. The NCI also suggests regular examinations for anyone with a large number of dysplastic nevi.

With new computerized technology, some dermatologists keep a digital photographic record of a patient's skin, which makes spotting changes in a mole much easier. They also use special magnifying instruments that allow them to see details in a mole that aren't obvious to the naked eye.

PREVENTIVE STRATEGIES

About 82 percent of melanomas are detected early, before they have a chance to spread. At this stage, they are highly curable. So performing a monthly skin self-exam, as described above, is an important step that does prevent invasive skin cancer. To find free professional skin cancer screenings in your community, visit the American Academy of Dermatology's Web site at www.aad.org.

On a day-to-day basis, the most important thing that you can do to prevent melanoma is to protect yourself from the sun. First and foremost, this means avoiding direct sun exposure between 10 A.M. and 4 P.M., when the ultraviolet radiation is most intense.

Although sunscreens are not proven to prevent melanoma, they can stop the severe, blistering sunburns that are known to increase melanoma risk. They also help protect against squamous cell skin cancers. So get in the habit of wearing a broad-spectrum, high-SPF sunscreen when you are outdoors. "Broad-spectrum" means that the sunscreen contains ingredients that block damaging UVA rays as well as burning UVB rays. According to one study, a high-SPF sunscreen that isn't broad-spectrum provides only half as much protection from immune-suppressing radiation as from sunburn. Look for products made with UVA blockers such as zinc or titanium and/or UVA absorbers such as Parsol 1789.

To remind people to safeguard their skin from the sun's harmful rays, the American Cancer Society uses the motto "Slip, Slop, Slap!" That is:

- Slip on a shirt with sleeves.

- Slop on sunscreen with an SPF of at least 15, and reapply every 2 hours.

- Slap on a wide-brimmed hat to shade your face, ears, and neck.

Research into how other lifestyle factors might influence skin cancer risk is limited at best. One study did show that regular exercise may help protect against melanoma. In this study, conducted at the University of Washington, men and women who worked out 5 to 7 days a week were less likely to develop melanoma.

With regard to diet, there is little evidence to suggest that any particular nutrient reduces skin cancer risk. A 2002 study of more than 5,000 women with basal cell skin cancer found that vitamins A, C, and E, folate, and carotenoids provided little protection against skin cancer. A 2003 study involving people with squamous cell skin cancer reached a similar conclusion. In fact, some researchers caution against taking supplements of antioxidants such as beta-carotene, since they may enhance the cancer process.

On the other hand, cutting back on dietary fat may have a protective effect. In a large Norwegian study of more than 50,000 people, a diet high in polyunsaturated fat was associated with an increased risk of melanoma in women, though not in men.

Another study examined the impact of diet on skin cancer patients with actinic keratoses, red, scaly patches that may develop into squamous cell carcinomas. Some of the patients limited their fat intake to just 20 percent of calories, while the rest followed a typical high-fat diet. After 4 months, those in the low-fat group had developed about three new actinic keratoses, on average. In the high-fat group, the average number of new lesions was 11.

Of course, more research is necessary to firmly establish a connection between dietary fat and skin cancer. But a high fat intake has so many other negative health implications that your best bet is to play it safe and curtail your fat consumption.

Dermatologists often recommend treatment for actinic keratoses not only because they are unattractive, itchy, and sometimes even tender but also because they can progress to squamous cell skin cancers. We don't know for certain how many lesions change in this way, but estimates range from 0.25 to 1 percent per year.

When a person has just a few actinic keratoses, a dermatologist may remove them by excision or with liquid nitrogen, which freezes them. The task is more challenging when a person has a number of lesions scattered across the skin's surface, including the forehead and arms. In this case, a doctor may choose to apply a medication such as topical 5-fluorouracil (5-FU) or diclofenac to the entire affected area. These medications are extremely irritating, which eventually causes the skin to peel—taking along with it the abnormal skin cells. The skin is red, mottled, and noticeably inflamed until healing is complete. By then many, if not all, of the actinic keratoses are gone, and the skin looks smooth and healthy.

Another treatment favored by some dermatologists involves applying aminolevulinic acid to a lesion, then activating the acid with a special light. Called photodynamic therapy, this treatment destroys the lesion quickly. But the activation process is uncomfortable, and may require anesthesia.

If you have actinic keratoses, you'll want to discuss all of these treatment options with your dermatologist. He or she can help weigh the pros and cons of each one, based on your particular situation.

CHEMOPREVENTION

Some provocative research with animals is looking into whether certain drugs, such as aspirin, could offset the cancer-causing effects of UV radiation. And one study involving humans suggests that regular use of aspirin and nonsteroidal anti-inflammatory drugs (NSAIDs) could reduce the risk of melanoma in women. Beyond that, though, we haven't seen a lot of evidence to support chemoprevention for melanoma.

In contrast, chemoprevention for nonmelanoma skin cancers is an active area of research. Currently, scientists are concentrating on two chemopreventive approaches: one involving tretinoin, which is a retinoid (a vitamin A derivative); the other using NSAIDs and celecoxib to block the COX-2 enzyme, which plays a role in the cancer process.

The FDA already has approved tretinoin to treat various skin conditions, including acne, sun damage, and age-related changes such as fine lines, roughness, and hyperpigmentation. Because tretinoin applied to the skin seems to improve or eliminate potentially precancerous actinic keratoses, scientists began to suspect that it might be an effective chemopreventive.

In 2002, a research team tested a topical retinoid, tazarotene, on mice that had been bred to develop basal cell skin cancers. The number of tumors in the animals declined by 85 percent. A clinical trial using tretinoin now is under way. The 1,200 participants—all with recent histories of nonmelanoma skin cancers—are applying either tretinoin or a placebo to their faces and ears twice a day. The objective of the trial is to determine whether the retinoid can curtail the appearance of actinic keratoses and the development of skin cancer.

The use of drugs to block the COX-2 enzyme and stop the process that leads to nonmelanoma skin cancers is especially exciting. Animal studies already have shown that the COX-2 inhibitor celecoxib not only reduces the number of tumors but also slows their formation. Now celecoxib is the focus of several clinical trials that are studying the effects of the drug in people with a genetic condition that predisposes them to basal cell skin cancers. It also is being tested as a treatment for actinic keratoses.

On the subject of actinic keratoses, another interesting development in chemoprevention for nonmelanoma skin cancers involves the topical application of imiquimod (Aldara) to the possibly precancerous skin lesions. Imiquimod is among a new class of drugs called immune response modifiers. Currently, it is approved as a treatment for genital warts.

When applied to the skin, imiquimod activates immune cells in the area, so they become extremely vigilant in recognizing and destroying abnormal cells—such as those in an actinic keratoses. Though imiquimod still is in the experimental stage, several reports suggest that using it three times a week for about 8 to 12 weeks can significantly reduce the number of precancerous lesions. The cream is irritating to the skin, so some people need to take a break of a few weeks between treatments. Whether or not imiquimod will be more effective than topical 5-fluorouracil remains to be seen.

WHAT YOU CAN DO NOW TO PREVENT SKIN CANCER

1. Examine your skin on a monthly basis.

2. If you notice any changes in a mole, report them to your doctor right away. Remember ABCDE: asymmetry, border irregularities, color variations, diameter larger than ¼ inch, and enlargement.

3. Ask your doctor to inspect your skin as part of your regular cancer checkup.

4. If you have a strong family history of melanoma, ask your doctor whether you should increase the frequency of your skin exams.

5. Protect yourself from the sun by applying a broad-spectrum, high-SPF sunscreen to your skin whenever you head outdoors. Wear protective clothing, including a hat that shades your face and ears.

6. Follow a healthy cancer-preventing lifestyle, which includes eating a low-fat diet and getting regular exercise.

CHAPTER 8

PROSTATE

CANCER

• • • • • • • • •

PROSTATE CANCER RANKS SECOND ONLY to skin cancer in the number of cases among men. Every year one in six men finds out he has this kind of cancer. For 2004, the American Cancer Society predicts that as many as 230,110 men will be diagnosed with the disease, and 28,500 will die from it.

African-American men are especially vulnerable to prostate cancer, for reasons that we still don't understand. The disease accounts for nearly 40 percent of all cancers that affect African-American men, with an incidence that is about 60 percent higher than for whites. In addition, African-American men are twice as likely to die from prostate cancer as American men from other ethnic groups.

While prostate cancer may hold the number two spot among causes of cancer death (lung cancer ranks first), about 98 percent of men who develop the disease survive for at least 5 years. That's because most prostate cancers—83 percent—are detected before they have spread, and they tend to grow slowly. As with other types of cancer, distinguishing prostate cancers that are aggressive and advancing rapidly from those that are unlikely to be life-threatening is an active area of research.

ARE YOU AT RISK?

1. ARE YOU OVER AGE 50? The incidence of prostate cancer increases with age, with 70 percent of cases occurring in men over 65. Since prostate cancer typically grows very slowly, one-third of men under 50 may have a precancer or very early stage cancer.

2. ARE YOU AFRICAN-AMERICAN? As mentioned above, African-American men have a higher incidence of prostate cancer than do men from other ethnic groups. They also tend to develop the disease at a younger age.

3. DO YOU HAVE A FAMILY HISTORY OF PROSTATE CANCER? Studies suggest that an inherited predisposition may be responsible for 5 to 10 percent of prostate cancers. The risk increases with the number of family members who have the disease. For example, if your father and brother have prostate cancer, you're two to three times more likely than the average man to develop the disease yourself. About half of prostate cancers that affect men under age 55 may result from an inherited prostate cancer susceptibility gene. But like most women with breast cancer, most men with prostate cancer show no family history of the disease.

4. DO YOU HAVE PROSTATIC INTRAEPITHELIAL NEO-PLASIA? Known as PIN for short, prostatic intraepithelial neoplasia involves an abnormal change in the tissue of the prostate gland ducts. Usually doctors find PIN when performing a biopsy because of suspected prostate cancer. PIN takes several forms. Those cases in which cells are very abnormal are known as HGPIN, with HG standing for high-grade. HGPIN is thought to be a prostate cancer precursor. The abnormal cells may appear in several areas of the prostate some 20 to 30 years before the onset of cancer. On the other hand, prostate cancer rarely occurs without HGPIN.

5. DO YOU FAVOR A HIGH-FAT DIET, WITH LOTS OF RED MEAT? Research indicates that while dietary factors like excessive fat consumption may not play much of a role in initiating cancer, they may accelerate the cancer process.

6. ARE YOU OVERWEIGHT? Research points to a conection between obesity and prostate cancer.

The Prostate Gland

BLADDER

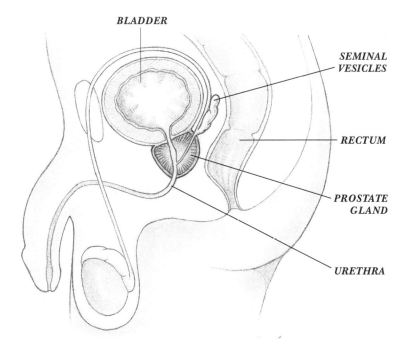

SEMINAL
VESICLES

RECTUM

PROSTATE
GLAND

URETHRA

THE PROSTATE IS ABOUT THE SIZE OF A WALNUT. IT SITS IN THE LOWER PELVIS LIKE AN UPSIDE-DOWN PEAR, COMPLETELY SURROUNDING A PORTION OF THE URE-THRA, THE TUBE THAT CARRIES URINE FROM THE BLADDER. THE PRIMARY PUR-POSE OF THE PROSTATE IS TO MANUFACTURE PROSTATIC FLUID, WHICH COMBINES WITH FLUID FROM THE SEMINAL VESICLES TO CARRY SPERM OUT OF THE BODY DURING EJACULATION.

THE PROSTATE CONSISTS OF GLANDULAR TISSUE, WHICH PRODUCES THE PROS-TATIC FLUID, AND MUSCLE, WHICH CONTRACTS DURING ORGASM TO FORCE SEMEN—A MILKY-WHITE MIX OF SPERM AND PROSTATIC FLUID—INTO THE URE-THRA. THE GLAND HAS THREE SECTIONS: THE PERIPHERAL ZONE, WHICH CON-TAINS MOST OF THE HUNDREDS OF GLANDS THAT SECRETE PROSTATIC FLUID; THE TRANSITIONAL ZONE, WHICH SURROUNDS THE URETHRA; AND THE CENTRAL ZONE, WHICH IS NEXT TO THE BLADDER. MOST CANCERS BEGIN IN THE PERIPHERAL ZONE, AND SOME IN THE TRANSITIONAL ZONE. RARELY DOES CANCER ORIGINATE IN THE CENTRAL ZONE.

7. ARE YOU SEDENTARY? Getting regular exercise is vital to maintaining a healthy body weight.

CAUSES

Like most cancers, prostate cancer probably arises from the convergence of several risk factors and triggers. By understanding how the cancer process unfolds, and identifying key turning points along the way, you stand the best chance of reducing your risk.

PROSTATE CANCER SUSCEPTIBILITY GENES. Research has yet to determine what damages the DNA of prostate cancer cells, permitting their uncontrolled growth. Scientists have succeeded in identifying several genetic mutations, known as prostate cancer susceptibility genes. These genes account for about 9 percent of all prostate cancers.

As with certain kinds of breast cancer, some—but not all—susceptibility genes associated with prostate cancer appear to be hereditary. We know of least six such genes so far. Recently, a gene associated with the process that causes hardening of the arteries was implicated in inherited prostate cancer as well. The gene, known as macrophage scavenger receptor-1 (MSR1), appears to participate in the body's inflammatory process.

Macrophages are white blood cells that rid the body of the debris that are by-products of infection. Researchers surmise that when the macrophage genes develop mutations, the cells can't do their job properly. This allows the buildup of debris, leading to inflammation of the prostate. One theory is that infection and inflammation may lead to prostate cancer.

In a 2002 study involving more than 700 men, about half of whom had prostate cancer, MSR1 mutations were seven times more common in those with cancer than in those who were cancer-free. Among the African-American study participants, 12.5 percent of those with cancer carried the mutations, compared with 1.8 percent of those who remained healthy. Despite statistics like these, acquired genetic mutations—that is, those that are not inherited—account for most prostate cancers.

Scientists also are looking into genes that could interact with certain environmental factors. For example, some genes are suspected of affecting hormone secretion, while others are involved in detoxifying pollutants. These kinds of genes may be responsible for many more prostate cancers than are the inherited susceptibility genes.

HORMONES. Research suggests that accumulated exposure to male hormones may raise the risk of prostate cancer. How androgens such as testosterone might contribute to cancer development remains to be seen. Studies have shown that when levels of androgens decline, the prostate becomes smaller, and levels of prostate-specific antigen (PSA) fall.

INSULIN-LIKE GROWTH FACTORS. Insulin-like growth factor-1 (IGF-1), which stimulates cell growth, may become a biomarker for prostate cancer if research can confirm that high levels are a reliable predictor of the disease. Studies to date have determined that men with high IGF-1 levels in their blood are four times more likely to develop prostate cancer than men with normal levels.

While the liver is responsible for producing insulin-like growth factors, other particulars—such as a person's nutritional status and circulating insulin level—appear to regulate just how much IGF-1 is in the bloodstream. In general, people who are overweight and sedentary tend to get higher IGF-1 readings.

DIETARY FAT. Ever since studies showed that the incidence of prostate cancer is lowest in countries like Japan, where the native population eats very little fat, scientists have been scrutinizing dietary fat as a contributor to the disease. Piquing their interest was the discovery that the incidence of prostate cancer appears to increase with each generation of Asians living in the United States. According to the National Cancer Institute, native Japanese have the lowest risk of prostate cancer, followed by first-generation Japanese-Americans, with an intermediate risk. Subsequent generations have the same risk as the general population of American men.

Research efforts to home in on the relationships between various types of dietary fat and prostate cancer have produced mixed and often contradictory results. According to one analysis, about half of the studies found an elevated cancer risk with increasing fat consumption, while the rest found no such correlation.

How might dietary fat affect the prostate? No one knows for sure. One theory is that certain fatty acids, such as the omega-6 fatty acids (linoleic acid), may stimulate cancer cells.

OCCUPATIONAL TRIGGERS. Exposure to dioxin—a contaminant from an herbicide used during the Vietnam War as well as in farming—is suspected of raising prostate cancer risk. So far, though, the research is inconclusive.

VASECTOMY. There has been some concern that vasectomy—a sterilization procedure that involves cutting the vas deferens—could raise prostate cancer risk. In fact, some urologists discourage men with a strong family history of the disease from undergoing the surgery. But a 2002 study from New Zealand, which has the highest rate of vasectomy in the world, found no correlation between the procedure and prostate cancer in men who were recently diagnosed with the disease.

SCREENING

According to current screening guidelines, physicians should offer annual tests for prostate abnormalities to all men ages 50 and older, as well as to younger men—ages 45 to 49—at high risk for prostate cancer. This includes African-Americans and anyone whose father or brother developed cancer at a young age. But the impact of these screening tests on early detection, and the benefit of early detection itself, remains controversial.

DIGITAL RECTAL EXAMINATION. In this screening test, known as DRE for short, a trained health care professional inspects the prostate by inserting a gloved finger into the patient's rectum and feeling for any hard or lumpy areas. For years DRE was the only available method of checking for prostate cancer. Unfortunately, it can easily miss a suspicious growth. Even today, scientists aren't sure whether annual DRE can reduce a man's chances of dying from prostate cancer.

PROSTATE-SPECIFIC ANTIGEN TEST. Prostate cells manufacture PSA, which then circulates in the bloodstream. If the gland becomes enlarged for any reason, it churns out even more PSA, raising the amount of the protein in the blood. Checking PSA levels involves a simple blood test. By repeating the test on an annual basis, you reduce your chances of missing even a slight upward spike in the protein.

The average man has a PSA reading between 0 and 4 nanograms per milliliter of blood (ng/ml). Between 4 and 10 ng/ml is slightly elevated, and between 10 and 20 ng/ml is moderately elevated. Anything above 20 ng/ml is considered highly elevated.

Keep in mind, though, that even a PSA level at the highly elevated end of the spectrum does not mean that you have cancer. In fact, the test often produces false-positive results, in which the protein appears to be abnormally high but no cancer is present. False-negative results, in which PSA measures are normal but cancer is present, also are common. According to several studies, about 65 percent of PSA tests are false positives, while at least 20 percent are false negatives.

So the first step after a PSA test in which the protein appears to be abnormally high is to repeat the test. If the PSA remains high, your doctor should recommend a more detailed workup. If this confirms an elevated PSA level, and if a digital rectal examination or a sonogram detects an abnormality, your doctor may want to do a biopsy. The procedure involves removing a tissue sample, usually through a needle, for microscopic analysis. But since so many factors can influence PSA—including infection, inflammation, benign prostate enlargement, and even age and race—most physicians won't perform a biopsy on the basis of one abnormal PSA test.

Routine PSA testing is controversial because it is not yet proven to save lives. Furthermore, a positive test result creates a dilemma for physician and patient alike. Because not all prostate cancers will progress, and not all will result in death, not all men require treatment. But obviously enough men are vulnerable—prostate cancer is, after all, the second most common cause of cancer deaths—that early detection is important.

To further complicate matters, even though an elevated PSA can lead to detection of a tumor so small that it probably would go unnoticed otherwise, there's no evidence that finding growths of such tiny size reduces a man's chances of dying from prostate cancer. Then, too, some tumors get so big so fast that they already have spread by the time they're detected.

Another consideration is that further diagnostic testing as a result of the elevated PSA can cause complications such as bleeding and infection. And if testing identifies the presence of cancer, surgery to remove the prostate can lead to impotence and incontinence.

In December 2002, the U.S. Preventive Services Task Force—a group of experts that sets policy for preventive health care—decided not to recommend for or against routine prostate cancer screening using digital rectal examination or PSA testing. Based on its review of the benefits and risks of screening, the USPSTF concluded that while PSA is more effective than DRE in detecting prostate cancer, no "good-quality evidence" proves that early detection would reduce the number of deaths from the disease. The task force did advise men to consult their personal physicians before deciding whether or not to undergo testing.

Currently, the National Cancer Institute is conducting the Prostate, Lung, Colon, and Ovarian (PLCO) Screening Trial, a randomized clinical trial involving more than 150,000 people. One of the research objectives is to determine whether the combination of annual digital rectal examination and PSA testing can reduce the number of prostate cancer deaths. The study will not conclude for several more years.

Separately, scientists are looking for ways to improve the accuracy and reliability of PSA testing. For example, measuring different types of PSA, rather than the total amount, might be a better predictor of prostate cancer. Some researchers believe that the test should account for changes in PSA with age, as what's "normal" varies according to how old a man is. Others think the test might be more accurate if it concentrated on sharp increases in PSA levels. Further research will help identify other biomarkers that may serve as more precise indicators of prostate cancer.

TRANSRECTAL ULTRASONOGAPHY. Although it is not a routine screening test, transrectal ultrasonography (TRUS) can help detect abnormalities in the presence of elevated PSA or confirm an abnormal area from a digital rectal exam. The test uses a thin probe inserted in the rectum to pick up sound waves as they bounce off the prostate. Then a computer converts the waves to an image.

Since normal tissue and tumors are distinctly different on a sonogram, many physicians rely on TRUS to guide them through a biopsy of the prostate. Studies show that the test may be more accurate in detecting prostate cancer than a random sample of prostate tissue.

PREVENTIVE STRATEGIES

While the exact role of dietary fat in prostate cancer remains a mystery, we think that limiting your fat intake—especially animal fat—is a wise move. Certainly, sticking with a low-fat diet has other health benefits, such as helping to maintain a healthy cholesterol profile, controlling your blood pressure, and protecting against both cardiovascular disease and colorectal cancer.

We know that Asian men—who tend to have a low incidence of prostate cancer—not only eat little animal fat but also consume up to 90 times as much soy foods, like tofu, soy milk, and miso, as their American counterparts. Certain components of soy may act as weak estrogens, inhibiting prostate cancer growth. Studies in this area focus on foods, not on specific micronutrients—an important distinction if you're thinking of trying these plant estrogens, or phytoestrogens, in supplement form.

Getting more fiber from whole grains and fruits might have a protective effect as well. The theory is that fiber binds to androgens as they pass from the liver into the intestine, preventing absorption of these male hormones and thus limiting the prostate's exposure to them.

Eating vegetables might help fend off prostate cancer, and not just because they supply fiber. In the Physicians' Health Study, researchers established a link between high blood levels of a nutrient called lycopene—the result of a high intake of tomatoes and tomato products—and a reduced risk of prostate cancer.

Several intriguing studies suggest that antioxidants like lycopene, vitamin E, and the trace mineral selenium help lower prostate cancer risk. We favor eating antioxidant-rich foods, primarily fruits and vegetables, to protect against all cancers. Don't rely on supplements to satisfy your antioxidant needs, at least until research proves that they are as effective as food sources and safe in high doses.

CHEMOPREVENTION

Right now, scientists are conducting about a dozen clinical trials to examine the use of hormones; drugs such as eflornithine, or DFMO; and dietary approaches to reduce prostate cancer risk. The two most important are the Prostate Cancer Prevention Trial (PCPT), which ended in summer 2003, and the ongoing Selenium and Vitamin E Cancer Prevention Trial (SELECT).

THE PROSTATE
CANCER PREVENTION TRIAL

The objective of this study, which involved 18,000 men over age 55, was to determine whether the drug finasteride—commonly prescribed for benign prostate enlargement—could prevent prostate cancer in healthy men. It did. (The study used a particular brand of finasteride called Proscar. The drug also is available in a lower dose as Propecia, which treats baldness.)

Finasteride works by blocking 5-alpha reductase, an enzyme that's necessary for the conversion of the male hormone testosterone into dihydrotestosterone (DHT). DHT stimulates prostate growth, and it may play a role in prostate cancer. From prior studies, the researchers knew that finasteride could inhibit the development of prostate cancer cells in the laboratory. They also knew that men with deficiencies in 5-alpha reductase don't get prostate cancer.

In this trial, the men who had taken finasteride every day for 7 years developed 25 percent fewer prostate cancers than the men who had taken a placebo. But the finasteride group also showed a higher percentage of aggressive or high-grade tumors—about 6.4 percent, compared with 5.1 percent in the placebo group.

Another concern was side effects. The men on finasteride were more likely to experience sexual problems while taking the drug. Between 5 and 13 percent of them reported erectile dysfunction and a loss of interest in sex. On the other hand, they experienced fewer of the urinary problems that commonly occur with aging, probably because the prostate gland had decreased in size.

This trial is important because it demonstrates that drugs can protect against prostate cancer. Although finasteride may not be the best choice for all men, some may benefit from it. We encourage you to discuss your options with your physician, especially if you are at very high risk for prostate cancer.

THE SELENIUM AND VITAMIN E CANCER PREVENTION TRIAL

SELECT is the first study to explore whether vitamin E or selenium—or both—can prevent prostate cancer. The study, which receives funding from the National Cancer Institute, also will determine whether either nutrient has any impact on lung and colorectal cancers.

Recruitment for SELECT began in 2001, with more than 400 medical centers throughout the United States, Puerto Rico, and Canada actively seeking 32,400 male volunteers—healthy White men age 55 or older and healthy Black men age 50 or older. To be eligible for the study, the men must have a normal digital rectal exam and a PSA level of 4 ng/ml or less.

Previous studies indicated that selenium and vitamin E can reduce the incidence of prostate cancer. For instance, one large Finnish study involving 29,000 male smokers examined the effects of beta-carotene and vitamin E on lung cancer. Neither nutrient prevented lung cancer, but the men who took vitamin E were 32 percent less likely to develop prostate cancer. In another study, this one involving 1,000 people, selenium didn't reduce the incidence of skin cancer. But it did lower the incidence of prostate cancer in men by 60 percent.

Once recruitment for SELECT wraps up, the researchers will assign all of the men to one of four groups, each of which will take two pills a day. One group will get 400 milligrams of vitamin E, plus a placebo that looks just like selenium. Another group will get 200 micrograms of selenium, plus a placebo that looks just like vitamin E. The men in the third group will take both selenium and vitamin E, while those in the fourth group will take two placebos that look like selenium and vitamin E.

When they first enroll in the study, and once a year thereafter, the men will receive a digital rectal examination and a PSA test. The also will complete questionnaires about their dietary habits and supplement use. The researchers will collect fingernail and toenail clippings from the men, to analyze for selenium. They will check blood levels of vitamin E as well.

SELECT will continue for another 12 years. To learn more about the study, go to the SELECT Web site at http://swog.org or visit the National Cancer Institute Web site at http://www.cancer.gov/select.

WHAT YOU CAN DO NOW TO PREVENT PROSTATE CANCER

1. Eat at least five servings of fruits and vegetables a day, and try your best to get nine.

2. Limit your consumption of red meat. And when you do eat meat, choose lean cuts and smaller portions.

3. Limit high-fat dairy products.

4. Increase your physical activity in all aspects of your life—on the job, at home, and in your leisure time.

5. Maintain a healthy weight for your size and build. As you grow older, you may need to reduce your calorie intake from food and increase your calorie burn through exercise in order to keep off any extra pounds.

6. If you smoke, stop.

7. Get an annual digital rectal examination and PSA test beginning at age 50, or age 45 if you are African-American or your father or brother has had prostate cancer.

CHAPTER 9

BREAST

CANCER

• • • • • • •

AMONG CANCERS THAT AFFECT WOMEN, breast cancer has held the number one spot for many years. It's far ahead of lung cancer, which ranks number two. In 2003, breast cancer accounted for 32 percent of cancer diagnoses among women, compared with 12 percent for lung cancer.

The American Cancer Society predicts that in 2004, 215,990 women will learn that they have invasive breast cancers. This figure does not include noninvasive, or in situ, breast cancers, which occur at a much lower rate, with an estimated 59,390 cases in 2004.

The good news in all of the statistics is that fewer women are dying from breast cancer. In fact, in 1987, breast cancer fell behind lung cancer as the leading cause of cancer deaths among women. Still, the number of deaths remains high, with the disease expected to claim the lives of as many as 40,580 women in 2004. (While breast cancer rarely affects men, it could account for as many as 1,450 cancer diagnoses and 470 cancer deaths among men in 2004.)

One possible explanation for the declining number of breast cancer deaths is the increasing availability of mammography, coupled with the growing awareness among women of the need for periodic mammograms. Consequently, we're able to detect breast cancer at an earlier stage, when most forms of the disease are more curable. The rise in mammography screening also is a likely explanation for the surge in the number of breast cancer diagnoses in the 1980s, when the incidence rate jumped by 32 percent.

Of course, improvements in treatment are another important factor in the gradually declining death rate. For example, the number of women who survive early, localized breast cancers for at least 5 years has increased from 27 percent in the 1940s to 97 percent today.

You probably are familiar with the statistic about the average woman's having a one-in-eight or one-in-nine chance of developing breast cancer. While these numbers are disconcerting, what most women don't realize is that they reflect cumulative risk over an entire lifetime—that is, from birth to age 85. Perhaps a more accurate way to assess risk is to compare the actual incidence of breast cancer among various age groups.

AGE	INCIDENCE
25–29	8.2 women per 100,000
40–44	120.1 women per 100,000
50–54	200.8 women per 100,000
65–69	352 women per 100,000

While breast cancer is as common among African-American women as among Caucasian women, African-Americans are less likely to be diagnosed with disease—yet more likely to die from it. The reason for the disparity remains uncertain. Some experts attribute it to socioeconomic factors. Others speculate that young African-American women may develop a more aggressive type of breast cancer, or they may not receive the best medical care.

Breast cancer also is the most common malignancy among Hispanic-American women, though both the incidence and death rate are declining. Hispanic women are about 30 to 40 percent less likely to develop breast cancer than non-Hispanics.

ARE YOU AT RISK?

1. ARE YOU OVER AGE 50? Age is the most important risk factor for breast cancer. About 77 percent of women who develop the disease are over age 50. Fewer than 20 percent are in their forties.

2. DO YOU HAVE A FAMILY HISTORY OF BREAST CANCER? In fact, most women who develop cancer do *not* have a family history of the disease. Fewer than 10 percent of cases are inherited. Nevertheless, if you have breast cancer in your family, you are at above-average risk.

3. HAS ANY MEMBER OF YOUR FAMILY, FEMALE OR MALE, BEEN FOUND TO CARRY A MUTATED BRCA1 OR BRCA2 GENE? If so, you have a 50 percent chance of inheriting the mutation, which means that you may want to consider genetic counseling and testing. Should testing reveal that you also carry the mutation, you have a 50 to 85 percent chance of developing breast cancer, as well as an increased risk of ovarian cancer. But remember that BRCA gene mutations account for just up to 10 percent of breast cancers. Most cases are sporadic—that is, they are not inherited.

4. HAS ANYONE IN YOUR FAMILY HAD OVARIAN CANCER? This could signal the presence of a BRCA gene mutation, which also raises breast cancer risk. With a BRCA2 mutation, the lifetime risk of ovarian cancer is 16 percent. It climbs as high as 40 percent with a BRCA1 mutation.

5. HAVE YOU HAD CANCER OF THE OVARY, UTERUS, OR COLON? Ovarian cancer slightly increases the risk of breast cancer, particularly in those who carry BRCA1 or BRCA2 gene mutations. The risk doubles with a personal history of uterine (endometrial) or colorectal cancer.

6. ARE YOU OF ASHKENAZI JEWISH HERITAGE? About one in every 40 Ashkenazi Jewish women carries a BRCA1 or BRCA2 gene mutation. A study involving more than 200 of these women—all of whom had breast cancer—found the mutation in 30 percent of those diagnosed before age 40. Among those over 40, the figure declined to 10 percent. Women of Ashkenazi Jewish descent can develop sporadic (non-inherited) breast cancers as well.

7. DOES YOUR MAMMOGRAM REVEAL THAT YOU HAVE DENSE BREASTS? While younger women normally have dense breasts, this tends to diminish with age as fat replaces some of the breast tissue. Still, some older women have dense breasts, which can make spotting abnormalities on mammograms more difficult.

8. HAVE YOU EVER HAD A BREAST BIOPSY THAT DETECTED ABNORMAL CELLS? This condition, known as atypical hyperplasia, raises the risk of developing breast cancer about fivefold. Fewer than 20 percent of women under age 50 undergo breast biopsies for benign breast disease, but studies show that those with such conditions are more likely to develop breast cancer. The biopsy itself doesn't increase risk. Rather, the fact that the procedure is necessary is a marker for what physicians call an active breast.

9. HAVE YOU ALREADY HAD BREAST CANCER? The risk of developing a new cancer in the same breast if you had a lumpectomy, or in the opposite breast, increases slightly each year.

10. HAVE YOU RECEIVED RADIATION THERAPY TO YOUR CHEST FOR ANY OTHER TYPE OF CANCER? Women who've undergone radiation therapy for Hodgkin's disease, for example, are significantly more likely to develop breast cancer. In fact, some experts recommend early mammography screening after Hodgkin's.

11. DID YOU BEGIN MENSTRUATING AT OR BEFORE AGE 12? Early onset of menstruation means longer lifetime exposure to estrogen, which could increase your risk of breast cancer.

12. DID YOU HAVE YOUR FIRST CHILD AFTER AGE 30? Never having children or giving birth at a later age nearly doubles the risk of breast cancer. (On the other hand, breastfeeding at any age lowers risk.)

13. ARE YOU TAKING ORAL CONTRACEPTIVES, OR HAVE YOU IN THE PAST? Although overall the incidence of breast cancer is not higher among women taking the Pill, the risk does rise slightly for young women, especially for those who went on oral contraceptives before age 21 and continued with it for more than 10 years. For women who carry BRCA1 gene mutations, taking the Pill also may increase risk.

14. DID YOU GO THROUGH MENOPAUSE AT OR AFTER AGE 51? Breast cancer risk rises by about 3 percent for each year of delayed menopause. "Delayed" means onset after age 51, the average age of menopause for women in the United States.

15. HAVE YOU USED HORMONE REPLACEMENT THERAPY, OR ARE YOU ON IT NOW? According to several studies, women who are on HRT for more than 5 years have a higher risk of breast cancer. The risk declines over time once HRT stops.

16. ARE YOU OVERWEIGHT? Women who gain weight after age 18 are twice as likely to develop breast cancer after menopause as women who maintain their weight throughout their lives. Regardless of when the extra pounds begin to appear, being overweight increases breast cancer risk. Where the body stores the extra fat can be a risk factor, too. For instance, research has shown that women whose waistlines exceed 36 inches are 34 percent more likely to develop breast cancer than those whose waistlines are less than 28 inches.

17. DO YOU DRINK MORE THAN TWO ALCOHOLIC BEVERAGES A DAY? Moderate alcohol consumption can cause a modest increase in breast cancer risk. With heavy drinking, defined as four or more alcoholic beverages a day, risk nearly doubles. Some researchers believe that even a small amount of alcohol—say, one drink a day—can elevate risk slightly, by about 3 to 4 percent. According to one analysis, the lifetime risk of breast cancer is 1 in 7 for heavy drinkers, 1 in 11 for nondrinkers.

RISK ASSESSMENT PROGRAMS

A doctor may use one of several different programs to evaluate a woman's breast cancer risk. These programs translate information about a woman's personal and family history into her odds of developing breast cancer within a certain time frame. They don't account for some of the risk factors mentioned above, such as delayed menopause or alcohol consumption—possibly because these criteria did not appear in the database from which the programs drew their information. The absence of certain

Comparing Risk Assessment Models

To evaluate your chances of developing breast cancer, your doctor likely will use one of two popular risk assessment programs: the Gail Risk Model or the Claus Risk Model. Each one considers a slightly different set of risk factors, as this chart shows. Keep in mind that both models appear most reliable for White women; neither has been validated for African-American women.

	GAIL MODEL	CLAUS MODEL
Description	Bases risk estimate on Breast Cancer Detection and Demonstration Project Data, a long-term study assessing risk factors, screening, and subsequent development of breast cancer	Bases probability of breast cancer on data from the Cancer and Hormone Study, a large study done in the 1980s by the Centers for Disease Control to determine the relationship between oral contraceptive use and breast, endometrial, and ovarian cancers
Factors considered	Current age Age at first menstrual period Age at first live birth Number of first-degree relatives with breast cancer Number of breast biopsies	Current age Number of first- and second-degree relatives with breast cancer and their ages at the time of diagnosis
Pros and cons	Hasn't been validated for women under age 20, minorities, or those who already have had breast cancer Doesn't account for ovarian cancer in the family, breast cancer in the father's family, or second-degree relatives with breast cancer May overestimate risk if mother or sister developed breast cancer when older Underestimates risk for women from families with inherited BRCA1 or BRCA2 gene mutations Overestimates risk in women who have had one or more breast biopsies	More applicable than the Gail Model to those who may inherit breast cancer

risk factors does not diminish the usefulness or accuracy of the programs.

The two most common risk assessment programs are the Gail Risk Model and the Claus Risk Model. Each has advantages and disadvantages. In our opinion, the Claus model is a better predictor of risk for women with strong family histories of breast cancer, while the Gail model is more suitable for women of average risk.

If you have had breast cancer, you already are at high risk for a recurrence, in which case neither of these risk assessment programs will provide you or your doctor with additional information. In fact, you already are a candidate for risk reduction therapies, which we'll discuss a bit later in the chapter.

According to the National Surgical Adjuvant Breast and Bowel Project (NSABP) Breast Cancer Prevention Trial, you also may be especially prone to breast cancer if your 5-year risk is equal to or greater than that of an average 60-year-old woman, according to the Gail model. All women 60 and older are at high risk, since age is the greatest single risk factor for breast cancer.

If you are at high risk for any reason, talk with your doctor about your options for preventing breast cancer, and for catching the disease in its earliest stages. For example, you could start mammography sooner, or get the screenings more frequently. You also may be a candidate for additional testing, such as breast sonography or magnetic resonance imaging (MRI) (more on these later). And in case your family history points to a possible BRCA gene mutation, your doctor may recommend genetic counseling and testing.

Risk assessment for breast cancer should be a standard component of the annual gynecologic exam. Make sure that it's part of yours. In our practices, we provide genetic counseling and testing for patients who need it. If your doctor doesn't, she should be able to offer a referral to a genetic counselor or center.

GENETIC RISK

Only about 1 in 100 people—1 percent of the general population—carries a genetic mutation that predisposes her to breast cancer. As mentioned earlier, the occurrence of these mutations is especially high in Ashkenazi

Jewish women. Mutations in the BRCA1 and BRCA2 genes are the most common; women who inherit a flawed form of either gene have a 50 to 80 percent chance of developing breast cancer sometime during their lives. (In men, a mutated BRCA2 gene is associated with breast cancer.)

Normally, the BRCA genes play a role in stopping the growth of abnormal cells. If the genes become damaged for any reason, they no longer can protect cellular DNA—which means they can't prevent abnormal cells from growing and dividing. This could set the stage for breast and ovarian cancers, and possibly for other forms of the disease, such as pancreatic cancer.

A doctor will use a special program to calculate a woman's chances of carrying a genetic mutation. If her risk is high, the doctor likely will recommend genetic counseling and testing. The test itself involves drawing a blood sample for laboratory analysis.

The BRCA1 and BRCA2 gene mutations are of greatest concern, since they account for about 85 percent of inherited mutations. But others can influence breast cancer risk as well. For instance, carrying a mutated p53 gene, which normally suppresses tumor cell growth, can raise a woman's risk by 1 percent. She also is more likely to develop a brain tumor or leukemia.

Right now, we don't have a reliable test for the p53 gene mutation, though one may be available in the future. And as studies of the human genome progress, scientists likely will discover other gene mutations with ties to breast cancer.

An inherited genetic predisposition to breast cancer influences the impact of other risk factors for the disease. Take age as an example. Women with inherited breast cancers usually get their diagnoses about 10 years earlier than women with sporadic (noninherited) breast cancers. What's more, some research suggests that women who carry the breast cancer genes may be more susceptible to the cancer-causing effects of radiation than women who don't. So far, the connection between the two has not been proven.

In 2003, the American Society of Clinical Oncology updated its genetic testing recommendations, expanding its list of hereditary syndromes that might predispose a woman to breast, ovarian, and colorectal cancers. According to the revised guidelines, anyone who is contemplating genetic testing must be fully informed of the pros and cons before making a decision. Genetic counseling should cover the implications of the test results as well as the benefits and limits of preventive strategies, among other topics.

The Breast

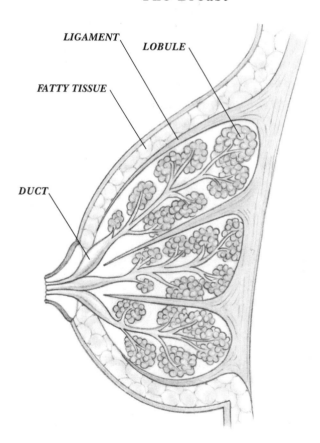

THE BREASTS CONSISTS OF MILK-PRODUCING GLANDS, OR LOBULES, SURROUNDED AND PROTECTED BY FATTY TISSUE AND LIGAMENTS. MILK FLOWS THROUGH SMALL DUCTS INTO LARGER AND LARGER ONES, FINALLY EMERGING FROM ONE OF SEVERAL DUCTS IN THE NIPPLE. MOST BREAST CANCERS BEGIN IN THE CELLS LINING THESE DUCTS.

CAUSES

All cancers are genetic in that they involve changes in DNA. But not all of these changes are inherited. Some result from so-called environmental factors. In cases of breast cancer, these factors can be both internal (fluctuating hormones) and external (poor diet). As we mentioned earlier in the chapter and throughout this book, age is the greatest risk factor for cancer, including breast cancer. This is because the older we get, the more vulnerable we are to the genetic mistakes that can increase our risk of the disease.

Some causes of genetic damage involve the risk factors listed above. But many more remain unknown. In fact, most women who develop breast cancer have no risk factors for the disease. This is not to minimize the value of assessing risk; on the contrary, if you know up front that you are at high risk, you can take control of the situation by adopting preventive measures and possibly stepping up breast cancer screenings.

From studies involving large numbers of women, we have learned that certain lifestyle choices affect the internal environment and may cause genetic damage, increasing breast cancer risk. We also know that some risk factors are not choices but still affect the internal environment. For instance, a woman can't do anything to change the age at which she began menstruating. If her first period appeared before she turned 12, she is more likely to develop breast cancer.

Researchers still are trying to understand and quantify the significance of certain environmental factors. One that has been the subject of considerable debate is a high-fat diet. An analysis of many studies throughout the world concluded that eating too much fat would raise the risk of breast cancer. Yet other studies in which researchers monitored the eating habits and health status of women over the course of many years found that dietary fat intake had no effect on breast cancer risk. Perhaps total calories and total body weight matter more.

Besides overweight and obesity, excessive alcohol consumption, radiation exposure, and hormone replacement therapy are known to contribute to breast cancer. So, too, may estrogen, as research has shown that women with breast cancer tend to have higher blood levels of the hormone than those who are cancer-free. Another hormone, progesterone, also may affect risk. Or perhaps both hormones working together is the real culprit.

We know for certain that having an increased number of menstrual cycles is a risk factor for breast cancer, which suggests some relationship between hormone levels and the disease. This is why early menstruation, delayed menopause, and no pregnancy can raise risk. On the other hand, breastfeeding helps lower risk, perhaps by reducing hormone levels or by stimulating the breast ducts to produce milk.

Smoking appears to play some role in breast cancer, though researchers are trying to determine just what that role might be. An analysis of studies conducted between the mid-1980s and 2000 identified a 10 percent increase in breast cancer risk among women who smoked, compared with those who never did. According to this analysis, the risk appeared highest just before women entered menopause, though it also was elevated in those who took up smoking at an early age.

Smoking may be particularly hazardous for women who are at high risk for breast cancer because of family history. Researchers at the Mayo Clinic Cancer Center found that among women with the highest genetic risk—that is, at least five cases of breast or ovarian cancer in their families—smokers were twice as likely to develop breast cancer as nonsmokers. Because this was a relatively small study, more research involving families with histories of the disease is necessary to determine just why smoking is so risky in these situations.

SCREENING

A number of screening tools and techniques can help spot abnormalities in the breasts in their earliest stages, when treatment is most effective. Perhaps the best known of these screening tests are the breast self-examination (BSE), in which you check for changes in your breasts and under your arms; clinical breast examination (CBE), in which a trained health professional inspects for abnormalities; and mammography, or breast x-ray. Physicians may supplement these with other tests, such as breast sonography and MRI—particularly if a suspicious area requires follow-up examination, if a woman has dense breasts, or if a woman is at high risk for breast cancer. Ductal lavage, though not appropriate for routine screening, also can be useful for those at high risk.

BREAST SELF-EXAMINATION

You have two good reasons to perform a breast self-exam on a monthly basis. One is to spot any lumps or irregularities that may indicate breast cancer. The other is to become familiar with your breasts so you will notice if anything suspicious does turn up. We tell our patients to perform

How to Examine Your Breasts

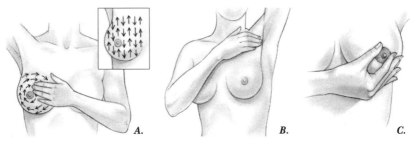

LIE ON YOUR BACK WITH A PILLOW UNDER YOUR RIGHT SHOULDER AND YOUR RIGHT ARM BE-HIND YOUR HEAD. USE THE FINGERS OF YOUR LEFT HAND TO PALPATE YOUR BREAST, VARYING THE PRESSURE AS YOU DO (A). REPEAT ON THE OPPOSITE SIDE. WHILE LYING DOWN, EX-AMINE THE CHEST AREA FROM EACH ARMPIT TO BENEATH EACH BREAST AND ALONG THE BREASTBONE TO THE COLLARBONE (B). ALSO CHECK EACH NIPPLE (C); IF YOU NOTICE ANY SECRETIONS, BE SURE TO REPORT IT TO YOUR DOCTOR.

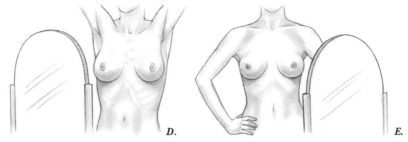

NEXT, STAND IN FRONT OF THE MIRROR WITH YOUR ARMS RAISED ABOVE YOUR HEAD. LOOK FOR IRREGULARITIES IN THE SHAPE, CONTOUR, OR COLOR OF YOUR BREASTS AND NIPPLES (D). REPEAT THE VISUAL EXAM WITH YOUR ARMS DOWN (E).

BSE right after their periods or, for menopausal women, once a month on their birth dates.

It's true that many breast lumps and abnormalities are caught by accident. It also is true that BSE can lead to unnecessary diagnostic testing, such as breast biopsy. And compared with BSE, mammography is far more likely to detect cancer. For all of these reasons, many experts have begun to question the value of BSE, leading to varying recommendations for breast self-exams.

We agree with the American Cancer Society's position that women should be informed about the benefits and limitations of BSE when they are in their twenties. They also should receive instruction in proper self-exam technique. In our practices, we teach BSE to our patients and then review it with them during their annual gynecologic exams.

We do encourage our patients to perform BSE, and we caution them not to panic if they find something suspicious. Most lumps and irregularities are not likely to be malignant. These days, we have breast sonography and other noninvasive tools that allow further evaluation of abnormalities, so biopsy—and the anxiety that accompanies it—may not be necessary (though for some patients, the alternative tools provoke anxiety, too).

CLINICAL BREAST EXAM

Whether women who have no symptoms of breast cancer should receive clinical breast exams on a regular basis also has generated some controversy. Data from studies analyzing the benefits and costs of CBE show that the screening plays only a minor role in cancer detection. Still, we share the American Cancer Society's opinion that until more conclusive research is available, CBE should remain part of a routine cancer checkup—preferably every year for women age 40 and older, and every 3 years for those in their twenties and thirties.

While annual mammograms also should begin at age 40 according to ACS guidelines, we believe that having a CBE when you see your doctor for your annual checkup is good supplemental insurance. Both of us have found breast cancer in patients with normal mammograms and no symptoms of the disease. If you or your doctor feels a lump, it requires further evaluation, even though your mammogram may suggest otherwise.

Ideally, you should schedule a CBE for after your period, when your breasts are less painful and "lumpy," and therefore easier to examine. Some experts recommend CBE shortly before a mammogram. This way, if your doctor notices anything unusual during his exam, he can adjust your mammogram to more closely inspect the suspicious area. Sometimes we prefer to schedule CBE and mammography 6 months apart so patients actually are getting screenings twice a year.

In our opinion, more studies are necessary before any decision is made to drop CBE from the annual cancer checkup. After all, research has yet to compare the outcomes of CBE with those of no screening. We remind our patients, too, that mammography is not 100 percent foolproof. Some cancers that don't show up on a mammogram can be seen or felt during a CBE or BSE.

In a study that ran from 1988 to 1991 and involved more than 2,000 breast cancer patients over age 50, 41 percent had found their tumors through mammography, and 11 percent with CBE. This percentage may seem comparatively small, but we believe it's high enough to justify a CBE at least once a year.

In our experience, monthly breast self-exam and annual clinical breast exam carry as much weight as mammography in the early detection of breast cancer. All three together are even more effective than just one or two in isolation.

MAMMOGRAPHY

Many screening guidelines have evolved from comparisons of mammography's lifesaving benefits versus its cost. These analyses tend to overlook one very important fact: Mammography can detect breast cancer at an early stage, when tumors are small and less aggressive therapy is a viable option. Research has shown that women between ages 50 and 69 benefit most from this screening—but even those under 50 are more likely to discover smaller tumors by having a mammogram than by waiting for the appearance of a lump.

The results of one fascinating study, published in the journal *Cancer* in 2003, offer even more evidence of the value of regular mammography for women in their forties. For the study, researchers reviewed the case histories of nearly 250 women who had developed breast cancer between ages 42 and 49. Among those who had not been getting screening mammograms, 52 percent already had advanced to a late stage of the disease by the time they were diagnosed, compared with 39 percent of those who had been getting mammograms at least every 2 years.

What this research suggests, simply stated, is that mammography can save lives, especially among women over age 40. This is why we advise our patients—as well as our family members, friends, and colleagues—to follow the American Cancer Society screening guidelines, which recommend that women at average risk for breast cancer get a mammogram every year beginning at age 40.

How long should you keep getting annual mammograms? This is an individual decision that should be based on your age, health, and life expectancy. In general, we think that as long as a woman is in good health, has a life expectancy of more than 3 to 5 years, and is willing to undergo treatment if she develops breast cancer, she should continue with her screenings.

Because the incidence of breast cancer is highest in older women, they especially should see their doctors for annual mammograms unless they have another serious illness that poses a more significant health threat. Unfortunately, many older women do not get this message. A study of more than 10,000 women in Michigan, all selected at random, determined that more than half of those over age 65 were not getting regular mammograms.

Looking ahead, a screening tool that soon may be getting more attention is digital mammography. Instead of using x-ray film, the device converts an image into digital format, which the doctor can magnify and manipulate to highlight specific areas. Digital images are easier to store, and they can be transmitted to other doctors via the Internet—provided, of course, that the new privacy provisions are followed.

A 3-year study of digital mammography—the Digital Mammographic Imaging Screening Trial (DMIST)—is under way at 35 medical centers across the United States and Canada. Its purpose is to compare digital imaging with traditional mammography to determine which is more accurate and cost-effective. The results of DMIST should be available in 2005.

We believe that digital mammography will compare favorably with standard mammography, and that the ease of storing and sharing the images may bolster its popularity. The downside is the cost of the equipment: Not all radiology facilities and hospitals will be able to afford it, and insurance may not cover the additional cost.

BREAST SONOGRAPHY

If a physician feels a lump in a patient's breast, he may use breast sonography, or ultrasound, to create images that will help determine whether the lump is a fluid-filled cyst or a solid mass. Ultrasound also can help clarify an abnormal area detected on a mammogram, and improve screening of dense breasts.

If a lump turns out to be a cyst, it probably is not malignant. A solid mass indicates the presence of a tumor, which generally requires biopsy— that is, the withdrawal of cells through a needle for microscopic examination. A biopsy also may be necessary in a situation where a mammogram is abnormal and the sonogram is normal.

Like mammography, breast sonography is a screening tool that detects abnormalities. It cannot *diagnose* cancer, since it doesn't extract a tissue sample for examination. One shortcoming of breast sonography is that unlike mammography, it cannot identify microcalcifications, or tiny calcified spots that may indicate cancer. While sonography will not replace mammography, it is very useful in certain situations.

IF YOU'RE AT HIGH RISK

In the late 1990s, a task force organized by the Cancer Genetics Studies Consortium made the following screening recommendations for women with BRCA1 or BRCA2 gene mutations:

- Monthly breast self-exam starting between ages 18 and 21
- Clinical breast examination every 6 to 12 months, starting between ages 25 and 35
- Annual mammography starting between ages 25 and 35

The task force also suggested that women who have strong family histories of breast cancer but who don't have the BCRA gene mutations begin annual mammography 5 to 10 years before the youngest age at which a relative developed the disease or at age 40, whichever is earlier.

The American Cancer Society has established slightly different screening guidelines for women at high risk for breast cancer. They include the following:

• Mammography screening beginning at age 30 or, in rare cases, younger

• Shorter intervals between mammography screenings, perhaps every 6 months

• Possible addition of breast sonography and/or MRI

If you suspect that you may be at high risk, according to the risk factors presented earlier in the chapter, talk with your physician about how often you should be getting mammograms and clinical breast exams. Also ask whether you might benefit from breast sonography or MRI.

Right now, the use of MRI as a breast cancer screening tool is relatively rare, though researchers are studying its effectiveness for women at high risk. Preliminary reports indicate that MRI is extremely sensitive in detecting abnormalities. But that could be a potential problem, as many of the abnormalities that show up during screening turn out to be benign. In the meantime, the patient may need to endure unnecessary diagnostic testing—and plenty of anxiety in the process.

A new screening technique that a growing number of doctors are using for women at high risk for breast cancer is ductal lavage. It involves retrieving fluid from the milk ducts for microscopic examination. This fluid contains mammary epithelial cells from the lining of the ducts. Most breast cancers begin in these cells. Some doctors describe ductal lavage as a "Pap smear for breasts" because the removal of cells to examine for abnormal changes is similar to the test for cervical cancer.

In general, the development of breast cancer takes years, during which the cells lining the milk ducts go through numerous changes. So the detection of precancerous abnormalities such as hyperplasia, which is an overgrowth of cells lining the ducts, can help keep the disease process from advancing too far. Likewise, catching very early stage cancers with a procedure like ductal lavage allows for treatment well before the disease turns invasive.

Before ductal lavage became available, evaluating cells from milk ducts in the nipple proved difficult. Usually it involved a procedure called fine-needle aspiration, which—as its name suggests—uses a needle to withdraw fluid directly from breast tissue. Because fine-needle aspiration is painful and yields few cells, doctors generally reserve it for when they already have found a mass through mammography, sonography, or clinical breast exam. In such cases, the needle is inserted directly into the suspicious area.

Another screening technique for cells from the milk ducts is nipple aspiration. In this procedure, a suction device is placed over the nipple to retrieve a small amount of fluid. Here again, the number of cells in the fluid tends to be low, which means identifying abnormalities and making an accurate diagnosis can be difficult.

Sometimes doctors "milk" the breasts by massaging them, then examine the cells in the fluid for suspicious changes. This screening technique does not deliver as many cells as ductal lavage.

Ductal lavage combines nipple aspiration with insertion of a very thin tube into a milk duct in the nipple. The aspiration process determines into which duct the tube should go. The doctor applies an anesthetic to the nipple to numb the area before gently threading the tube into the duct. An injection of saline solution into the tube rinses out the duct. Then the doctor withdraws the saline, which contains cells from the lining of the duct.

Ductal lavage is a promising screening technique. In one study involving more than 500 women, ductal lavage yielded 13,500 mammary epithelial cells for each duct, compared with 120 cells obtained through nipple aspiration or breast massage.

We perform ductal lavage on our patients who are at high risk for breast cancer as a means of further evaluating their risk. We view the procedure as a complement to clinical breast exam and mammography, in that it gives us a more complete picture of what is going on inside a woman's breast.

PREVENTIVE STRATEGIES

Some of the recommendations in this section, especially those pertaining to lifestyle factors, come from studies that have analyzed certain aspects of life—like diet and exercise—in large groups of women. These observational studies, as they are known, can identify and quantify an association between a particular risk factor and incidence of breast cancer, providing important clues to what sorts of measures may help protect against the disease. Bear in mind, these studies will not prove that a particular risk factor causes cancer, or that changing a certain behavior will reduce your risk.

In 1998, a team of Swedish and American scientists published their findings from an observational study of more than 6,000 women, providing strong evidence that women who once were lean but have gained weight are at highest risk for breast cancer. From similar research, we have learned that obesity raises the risk of breast cancer in older women, and that thinner women have a higher risk of breast cancer before menopause than after.

Several important studies now under way will yield a great deal of helpful information about the relationship between body weight, nutrition, and breast cancer risk. Among them is the Women's Healthy Eating and Living Study, which is examining the effects of a low-fat diet that includes five servings of fruits and vegetables a day in more than 3,000 women who've undergone treatment for early-stage breast cancer. Meanwhile, the much smaller Healthy Weight Management for Breast Cancer Survivors Study is exploring the impact of several factors, including diet and exercise, on breast cancer recurrence. And the Women's Intervention Nutrition Study is evaluating 2,500 women within a year of surgery for early-stage breast cancer to determine whether limiting dietary fat intake to no more than 15 percent of daily calories affects survival rate.

Of course, we can't automatically apply research findings from women who have undergone treatment for breast cancer to women who are healthy, even if they are at high risk for the disease. More research is necessary to determine whether the same factors have the same impact in both groups.

One of the largest research projects is the Women's Health Initiative, which is studying the incidence of breast and colorectal cancers, as well as other chronic diseases, in women ages 40 and older. The researchers hope to draw some conclusions about the influence of several lifestyle factors on cancer, such as following a low-fat diet rich in fruits, vegetables, and grains and using hormone replacement therapy.

Based on what studies have shown us so far, we can draw some reasonable conclusions about strategies that could help lower the risk of breast cancer, not to mention other forms of cancer. Here's what we recommend.

MAINTAIN A HEALTHY BODY WEIGHT. Without a doubt, being obese raises the risks of several types of cancer. Scientists don't yet know exactly how this happens, but they do have several theories. One is that since fat plays a role in the metabolism of estrogen, carrying too many fat cells provides a constant source of the hormone. And if cancer cells that are sensitive to estrogen happen to be present in the breast, the hormone will stimulate their growth.

In fact, some scientists speculate that estrogen may set the stage for breast cancer by accelerating cell division. Cells that divide rapidly are more susceptible to mistakes or mutations.

Whatever mechanisms may be involved, the relationship between obesity and breast cancer appears quite complicated. We still need to determine whether risk is driven by the amount of fat, the location of fat, or total body weight—or perhaps a combination of all three. Still, we have enough evidence from all those observational studies to recommend maintaining a healthy body weight as a strategy to protect against breast cancer. We strongly advise our patients to monitor their weight and to lose any extra pounds by watching their calorie intakes and increasing their activity levels. (For more advice on slimming down, as well as guidelines for determining your healthy weight, see page 223.)

BUILD YOUR DIET AROUND A VARIETY OF NUTRITIOUS FOODS. In 1998, *The Breast Cancer Prevention Diet* made the best seller lists by promising to reveal "the powerful foods, supplements and drugs that can save your life." The book stresses the importance of eating more fruits and vegetables, getting adequate amounts of key nutrients and fiber, and controlling weight. Still, many women assumed from the cover that certain foods, like soy, or specific nutrients, like omega-3 fatty acids or vitamin D, could stop breast cancer. The reality, of course, is not that simple.

Take dietary fat as an example. Eating too much of it is unhealthy for a lot of reasons—not the least of which is that gram for gram, fat contains more calories than other nutrients. What's more, a high fat intake is a known risk factor for breast cancer in postmenopausal women. But despite efforts to find an association between total dietary fat or even specific types of dietary fat and breast cancer, scientists have not been able to confirm such a link.

Nor have they found conclusive evidence that eating meat, a major source of fat in the typical American diet, can raise the risk of breast cancer. In fact, a very large analysis of data from more than 27,000 vegetarians and nearly twice as many nonvegetarians found no difference in risk.

While studies have not proven that dietary fat is a crucial player in the cancer process, the question remains open to debate. Several studies currently under way finally may settle the issue. The Women's Intervention Nutrition Study, for example, may reveal important information about the value of following a low-fat diet because some of the participants are restricting their fat intakes to 15 percent of their total calories.

Even as we await the findings of these studies, we are advising our patients to follow the American Cancer Society dietary guidelines, which recommend choosing low-fat foods and limiting red meat, especially fatty cuts. We also stress how focusing on just one nutrient or one food is not the healthiest dietary approach for cancer prevention. Eating a variety of foods while keeping an eye on calories makes much more sense.

So what about those "powerful foods"? Soy has received a great deal of attention in the popular press because it contains high levels of phyto-estrogens. These are plant substances that attach to hormone receptors in the body, turning on or off cellular activities that rely on estrogen.

In Asian countries where soy and soy products are dietary mainstays, the incidences of both breast and prostate cancers are low. Of course, other aspects of the Asian lifestyle are different, too. But since soy contains substances that act like estrogen, many experts suspect that eating large quantities of soy helps prevent breast cancer. It's a logical assumption, but not a proven one, as studies in Asian countries have failed to find any association between soy and reduced breast cancer risk. Indeed, some studies suggest that too much soy actually may increase risk.

Eating too many soy foods isn't easy. But the growing availability of soy powders and pills has made excessive consumption a serious concern. We advise against using these supplements. Lowering breast cancer risk through diet means eating whole foods, not taking separate micronutrients in pills or powders.

After all, soy contains many compounds besides phytoestrogens that do not act like hormones. In animal studies, these compounds appear to affect cancer cells. Eventually research may prove that soy is a powerful anticancer food, but today all we know is that soybeans—like any bean (such as chickpeas) and in any form (such as tofu)—are a smart choice for a healthy diet.

LIMIT YOUR ALCOHOL CONSUMPTION. The evidence linking alcohol to breast cancer is fairly conclusive. Even having just a few drinks a week appears to raise risk. This has prompted the American Cancer Society to recommend that women limit themselves to one drink a day—the equivalent of 12 ounces of beer, 5 ounces of wine, or 1½ ounces of 80-proof distilled spirits.

Scientists still aren't sure how alcohol contributes to the cancer process. Studies have shown that women with high estrogen levels consume about three times as much alcohol per week as women with low estrogen levels, which suggests that alcohol could elevate the hormone. It also may deplete folic acid, which offers some protection against cancer.

Yet another possibility is that once in the body, alcohol breaks down to form chemicals that affect breast tissue.

INCREASE YOUR ACTIVITY LEVEL. A physically active lifestyle can reduce breast cancer risk by 10 to 25 percent, though just what drives this protective effect remains unknown. The theory is that as long as exercise is vigorous but not exhausting, it enhances immune function. A healthy immune system can help fend off a host of diseases, including many kinds of cancer.

Exercise also may contribute to breast cancer prevention by building lean muscle mass. This is important for maintaining a healthy body weight; for reducing body fat, a source of estrogen; and for inhibiting estrogen production.

In 2000, Dutch researchers published a study comparing the exercise habits of nearly 1,000 women ages 20 to 54 who had invasive breast cancer, and an equal number of women who were cancer-free. The researchers identified a 30 percent reduction in breast cancer risk among the healthy women who were physically active. Consistency of physical activity and weight control appeared to be key factors. The researchers reported that women who engaged in exercise on a regular basis and maintained healthy weights for their heights experienced the greatest protective effect.

In this study, exercise appeared to have a positive impact on risk no matter what a woman's age when she began working out consistently. Interestingly, though, the women who were physically active before age 20 seemed more likely to remain active throughout life. Being active from an early age may help reduce the risk of breast cancer by delaying the onset of menstruation.

Later in 2000, a study involving thousands of women in the United States concluded that the most dramatic reduction in breast cancer risk occurred in women who had engaged in some form of strenuous physical activity at least once a day early in their lives. What's more, active women who had lost weight or had gained only a small number of pounds over the years were half as likely to develop breast cancer after menopause as inactive women who had not gained weight.

This research supports the theory that building lean muscle mass, minimizing body fat, and maintaining a healthy body weight can help protect against breast cancer. It becomes even more important with age because the natural tendency is to do just the opposite—that is, lose muscle mass and increase body fat. So even if you maintain a healthy body weight, you need to be careful to avoid an unhealthy shift in body composition. And the best way to do it is to increase your activity level.

A year after these studies were published, the International Agency for Research on Cancer of the World Health Organization held a conference in Lyon, France, for a group of international experts. After reviewing the literature on weight control and physical activity in cancer prevention, they concluded—among other things—that sufficient evidence exists in favor of physical activity to protect against breast and colorectal cancers. Incidentally, more recent research suggests that remaining active in all aspects of your life—on the job, at home, and in your leisure time—throughout your life reduces your risk of breast cancer after menopause.

PREVENTIVE SURGERY

Now that genetic testing for breast cancer is available, women who learn that they inherited BRCA1 or BRCA2 gene mutations—and who therefore have a 50 to 90 percent chance of developing breast cancer—must make some difficult decisions. Most choose closer surveillance, which means starting mammograms at an earlier age, getting regular clinical breast exams, and doing regular breast self-exams. Some opt to take a chemopreventive drug such as tamoxifen (which we'll discuss in just a bit). And some decide to undergo a bilateral prophylactic mastectomy, which involves removing all the tissue of both breasts, including the nipples. The muscle beneath the breasts remains intact, as do the lymph glands under the arms. Many women who choose this procedure undergo breast reconstruction at the same time or shortly thereafter, using either their own tissue or breast implants.

Understandably, many women are reluctant to pursue such drastic surgery, even when they carry the BRCA1 or BRCA2 gene mutations. After all, breasts play an important role in a woman's body image, helping to shape not only her sexuality but also her feminine identity. What's more, breasts are essential for those women who are contemplating pregnancy and wish to breastfeed their newborns.

So while prophylactic mastectomy is right for some women, those who don't feel comfortable with it have alternatives for reducing their risk of breast cancer, such as taking tamoxifen. If you are weighing this decision, keep in mind that the surgery produces a nearly 90 percent drop in risk, compared with about 50 percent for tamoxifen.

Prophylactic mastectomy also is an option for women who have had cancer in one breast and who have family histories of the disease. For these women, the odds of developing cancer in the opposite breast within 16 years of the first diagnosis are 35 percent. The risk is just 1 percent for women who've had cancer but who don't have family histories. Not long ago, a study from the Mayo Clinic concluded that prophylactic mastectomy of the opposite breast reduces the chances of recurrent breast cancer by 94.4 percent.

Women who carry the BRCA1 or BRCA2 genetic mutations should also discuss prophylactic oophorectomy with their physicians. Research has shown that among women in this group who are premenopausal, the risk of breast cancer falls by about 30 to 50 percent if their ovaries are removed before age 50. This is because without their ovaries, they stop producing estrogen. (To learn more about prophylactic oophorectomy, see chapter 12.)

In the late 1990s, the group of experts who comprise the Cancer Genetics Studies Consortium met to come to a consensus on guidelines for women who inherit BRCA1 or BRCA2 gene mutations. They recommended early breast and ovarian cancer screenings for those with BRCA1 gene mutations, and early breast cancer screenings for those with BRCA2 mutations. They took no position on prophylactic surgery. You should be aware, though, that the consortium developed these guidelines prior to the NSABP Breast Cancer Prevention Trial and prior to the availability of data showing the effectiveness of prophylactic surgery for women at high risk for breast cancer.

TAMOXIFEN

In 1998, the Food and Drug Administration approved tamoxifen (Nolvadex) as a preventive for breast cancer—the first-ever drug to earn this distinction. According to the FDA, physicians may prescribe tamoxifen to women over age 35 who have a predicted 5-year breast cancer risk of at least 1.67 percent according to the Gail model. For instance, a young woman who has been diagnosed with ductal carcinoma in situ (a tiny cancer that develops in the breast duct and may not become invasive)or whose mother had breast cancer might be a candidate for tamoxifen therapy. We also recommend tamoxifen to our patients who carry the BRCA1 or BRCA2 gene mutations, though currently data assessing the drug's protective effect are not as strong for women with BRCA1 mutations as for those with BRCA2 mutations.

Since researchers have not studied tamoxifen use by women with an average risk of developing breast cancer, the FDA has not approved the drug for this purpose. It might not improve risk for these women, and it might expose them to potentially harmful side effects. Most of these side effects, such as hot flashes and vaginal dryness, are annoying but manageable. But some are serious enough that they restrict who can use tamoxifen therapy. For instance, women with a history of clotting problems or precancerous conditions of the uterus should not take the drug. Nor should women who are breastfeeding or who want to become pregnant. Tamoxifen can affect fertility and may cause birth defects.

With tamoxifen, the balance between risk and benefit varies from one woman to the next. Even for the same woman, the nature and intensity of side effects may change over time. That is why discussing this chemopreventive therapy with your physician, and even getting a second opinion, is so important.

In our opinion, the results of randomized clinical trials make it clear that tamoxifen prevents breast cancer and saves lives. But the drug also presents a very real risk of side effects, most commonly in women over age 50. For this reason, it seems to us that the ideal candidate for tamoxifen therapy is a woman who is between ages 35 and 50 and at high risk for breast cancer, unless she has undergone a hysterectomy, in which case she could continue therapy until age 65.

In 2002, the American Society of Clinical Oncology (ASCO) reviewed the available literature and heard expert opinions about chemoprevention for breast cancer. The final conclusion of this investigation was similar to the FDA-approved indication for tamoxifen. Specifically, the ASCO Cancer Technology Assessment Working Group concluded that "for women with a 5-year projected breast cancer risk greater than 1.66 percent, tamoxifen 20 milligrams daily for 5 years may be offered to reduce their risk." Even if therapy stops after 5 years, the drug's protective effect appears to last for another 5.

In spring 2003, a study published in the *Journal of the National Cancer Institute* revealed that even though 10 million women are eligible for treatment with tamoxifen, which would cut their risk of breast cancer by half, only about 500,000 are taking it. And most of them are taking it because they already have had breast cancer. Even after eliminating those women who are at risk for serious side effects, it leaves some 2.47 million who could benefit from tamoxifen therapy. Experts speculate that if all of these women were to take tamoxifen for 5 years, it could prevent or delay more than 28,000 breast tumors.

The obvious question is, why are so many women not taking tamoxifen? In our opinion, one major barrier is an unrealistic concern about potential side effects. Reports from the NSABP Breast Cancer Trial about side effects were unnecessarily alarming because of how they were interpreted. For instance, one report noted that women who took tamoxifen were more likely to develop a blood clot in the lung than those who took the placebo. The actual numbers paint a very different picture: Of 7,000 women, 30 developed blood clots—but only 18 in the tamoxifen group, compared with 12 in the placebo group.

In much the same way, the risk of uterine cancer with tamoxifen therapy seems to have been misconstrued. The researchers counted 15 more cases of uterine cancer among the women on tamoxifen than among those taking a placebo. But for a group of 7,000 women, the actual risk seems comparatively small.

Of course, every woman who is considering tamoxifen therapy should undergo careful evaluation with regard to several factors, including her current health status, her risk of developing breast cancer, her risk for other conditions such as uterine cancer and blood clots, and her willingness to be monitored for side effects. But unrealistic fears of possible side effects should not interfere with the use of this chemopreventive drug.

CHEMOPREVENTION

The NSABP Breast Cancer Prevention Trial found 49 percent fewer breast cancers among the women who took tamoxifen than among those who took the placebo. At the end of the trial, those in the placebo group were given the option of switching to tamoxifen or joining an ongoing trial known as STAR, for the Study of Tamoxifen and Raloxifene.

Like tamoxifen, raloxifene is a SERM—short for selective estrogen receptor modulator. (For further information on how SERMS help protect against cancer, see chapter 6.) In 1997, the FDA approved raloxifene (Evista) to prevent osteoporosis in women who have gone through menopause. When a study identified a 70 percent reduction in breast cancer risk among women taking raloxifene compared with those taking a placebo, researchers became cautiously optimistic about using the drug for chemoprevention. The caveat with these findings is that the women who participated in the study, called MORE (Multiple Outcomes of Raloxifene Evaluation), had shown a lower-than-average breast cancer risk even before they even went on raloxifene.

Some experts believe that raloxifene may have less powerful antiestrogen activity in the breast and uterus than tamoxifen does. So raloxifene could turn out to be as effective in preventing breast cancer, but less likely to cause uterine cancer. On the other hand, it may turn out to be less effective in preventing breast cancer in women at high risk for the disease. We won't know until the STAR trial is complete.

Among the women in the MORE trial, a larger number of those taking raloxifene were more likely to develop blood clots than were those taking a placebo. So this side effect remains a concern, just as it is for tamoxifen and hormone replacement therapy. Raloxifene is known to cause some minor side effects as well, including hot flashes and vaginal discharge, dryness, or itching.

The STAR trial aims to answer questions about how tamoxifen and raloxifene compare in terms of short-term and long-term safety and effectiveness. Recruitment for the trial—the largest ever to focus on breast cancer prevention—began in 1999, with researchers hoping to find 19,000 volunteers at 500 medical centers across the United States, Puerto Rico, and Canada. To be eligible for the trial, a women must be at least 35 years old; already have gone through menopause; and show a breast cancer risk equal to but no greater than the average woman between ages 60 and 64 or a Gail model score above 1.7.

The researchers randomly assign the women to take either 20 milligrams of tamoxifen or 60 milligrams of raloxifene every day for 5 years. Neither the women nor their doctors know which drug they're taking. During the course of the trial, the women will receive regular mammograms and gynecologic exams. Preliminary results should be available in 2005.

Besides tamoxifen and raloxifene, new SERMs are in the pipeline. So you're likely to be hearing even more about this class of chemopreventive drugs in the future.

CELECOXIB TRIAL

Several studies have indicated that certain nonsteroidal anti-inflammatory drugs (NSAIDs), which block production of an enzyme called cyclooxygenase (COX), can help protect against breast cancer. In fact, regular use of NSAIDs is associated with an estimated 18 percent reduction in breast cancer risk.

A clinical trial currently under way at four medical centers is investigating whether celecoxib (Celebrex), a prescription COX-2 inhibitor, might help prevent breast cancer. All of the study participants have inherited BRCA1 or BRCA2 gene mutations, but none has gone through menopause. They will take celecoxib twice a day for 1 year. After that, their doctors will remove fluid from their breasts, using either ductal lavage or fine-needle aspiration, to check for abnormal cells. They will repeat the test every year for 5 years.

In 2003, researchers released an analysis of data from the Women's Health Initiative with the conclusion that women who had taken aspirin and ibuprofen (which block both COX-1 and COX-2) at least every other day for 5 to 9 years were 21 percent less likely to develop breast cancer than women who hadn't taken the drugs. This finding adds to the body of evidence suggesting that blocking the COX enzyme may be an effective approach to lowering breast cancer risk. The celecoxib trial could help determine whether further study of NSAIDs is necessary.

Although this is very exciting research, we are not yet recommending aspirin or ibuprofen therapy to our patients at high risk for breast cancer. Regular use of either drug can cause side effects.

BEXAROTENE TRIAL

Studies using bexarotene (Targretin), a vitamin A derivative, to treat breast cancers in laboratory animals have shown that many of the cancers regress. Other research has concluded that bexarotene is helpful for women with breast cancer that has spread. Now researchers at Baylor College of Medicine are conducting a clinical trial to see whether bexarotene might help prevent breast cancer.

For this trial, all of the volunteers must be at high risk for breast cancer. Women are not excluded if they had the disease in the past. But they must have completed chemotherapy at least a year before, and tamoxifen therapy at least 3 months before.

INDOLE-3-CARBINOL

Natural substances called indoles may be responsible for the cancer-fighting properties of cruciferous vegetables. But the very thought of eating large quantities of broccoli and cabbage won't appeal to everyone. This has prompted researchers to see whether they can isolate one of these powerful antioxidants—like indole-3-carbinol—and package it in pill form.

While animal studies have shown that large doses of indoles can reduce breast tumors, human research is at a preliminary stage. Furthermore, other studies have suggested that taking supplements of single micronutrients actually may raise cancer risk. Until we know more, we don't recommend any supplements other than a daily multivitamin.

The first phase of a study to examine the safety of indole-3-carbinol for women at high risk for breast cancer is under way at the University of Kansas Medical Center. Other research has investigated whether the micronutrient might help prevent cervical cancer. While the early studies were encouraging, placebo-controlled trials were not.

What You Can Do Now to Prevent Breast Cancer

1. At your next annual gynecologic exam, ask your doctor to calculate your breast cancer risk. Several Web sites now offer risk assessment calculators; one is www.breastcancerprevention.com, the official Web site of the NSABP Breast Cancer Prevention Trial.

2. If you are at average risk, do a breast self-exam every month, ideally starting at age 20. Follow up with a clinical breast exam at least every 3 years between ages 20 and 39, then every year starting at age 40. Also get a mammogram every year starting at age 40.

3. If you are at high risk, talk with your doctor about which screening tests you need and at what intervals.

4. If you are at high risk, ask your doctor whether you'd be a candidate for tamoxifen therapy. Or you may want to consider enrolling in a clinical trial of another chemopreventive drug.

5. Make every effort to maintain a healthy weight. As you get older, this may mean eating fewer calories and getting more exercise.

6. Eat at least five servings fruits and vegetables a day, and do your best to get nine.

7. Find ways to become more physically active in every aspect of your life—on the job, at home, and in your leisure time.

8. If you smoke, stop.

9. If your mother, sister, or daughter has breast cancer, seek genetic counseling before deciding whether to undergo genetic
   testing.

10. If genetic testing reveals that you carry the BRCA1 or BRCA2
    gene mutation, talk with your doctor about your options for
    managing your breast cancer risk. You could take tamoxifen or
    enroll in a clinical trial. Another possibility is preventive surgery
    (prophylactic mastectomy and/or oophorectomy).

CHAPTER 10

L U N G

C A N C E R

• • • • • • •

THE INCIDENCE OF LUNG CANCER IN THE U.S. population kept climbing year after year for decades. Finally, in the 1990s, the upward trend began to level off as new cases among men dropped significantly and new cases among women reached a plateau. That's the good news.

The bad news is that the incidence of lung cancer remains very high. It ranks as the second most common cancer diagnosis among men and women, and it's the leading cause of cancer deaths in the United States and throughout the world. In the late 1980s, it surpassed breast cancer as the leading cause of cancer death among women. The death rate from lung cancer continues to rise among African-American women, probably because they are a bit behind men in giving up smoking.

This is the real tragedy of lung cancer: It would be almost entirely preventable, if only people would stop smoking. Although half of all living Americans who ever smoked have quit, as many as 46.5 million— nearly one-quarter of the population—still light up.

And so we continue to see grim statistics like these. In 2004, a predicted 13 percent of all diagnosed cancers will be lung cancers, affecting 173,770 people. According to experts, as many as 160,440 will die from the disease.

One reason lung cancer is so deadly is that early diagnosis is so difficult. Only 15 percent of lung cancer patients are in the early stages of the disease. The overall cure rate is just 10 percent.

If you were to look at a graph with lines to represent the average number of people who smoke and the average number who die from lung cancer, you would see that the decline in death rate lags several decades behind the decline in the smoking population. In 1963, for example, more Americans than ever were smoking. About 25 years later, the number of men dying from lung cancer reached a peak. The peak in the death rate among women didn't occur for another decade. This is because women took up smoking about 20 years later than men, and they quit later—that is, at least until the mid-1980s. Their death rate from lung cancer finally began to fall in the early 1990s.

Just as there are differences between genders in smoking habits and lung cancer rates, so are there differences between ethnic groups. For instance, lung cancer rates are about 40 percent lower among Hispanics than among other groups. Not coincidentally, Hispanics also are less likely to smoke.

ARE YOU AT RISK?

1. DO YOU SMOKE? More than 87 percent of lung cancer cases are a direct result of smoking.

2. DID YOU EVER SMOKE? It's true that compared with those who continue smoking, those who have been smoke-free for more than 10 years are half as likely to develop lung cancer. Still, the longer you smoked, the more damage you did to your lungs. Former smokers account for about half of all new lung cancer cases each year.

3. DO YOU LIVE WITH A SMOKER? If so, your risk of lung cancer is about 35 to 53 percent higher than that of someone who lives with a nonsmoker. We know that spouses of smokers are 30 percent more likely to develop lung cancer than spouses of nonsmokers.

4. ARE YOU EXPOSED TO SECONDHAND SMOKE AT WORK? The toxic smoke comes not only from the lit cigarette, cigar, or pipe but also from the smoker, who exhales it into the air you breathe.

Depending on your situation, you may be exposed to more smoke at work than at home.

5. ARE YOU MIDDLE-AGED OR OLDER? The average age for lung cancer diagnosis is 60. Like most other cancers, lung cancer develops over many years.

The Lungs

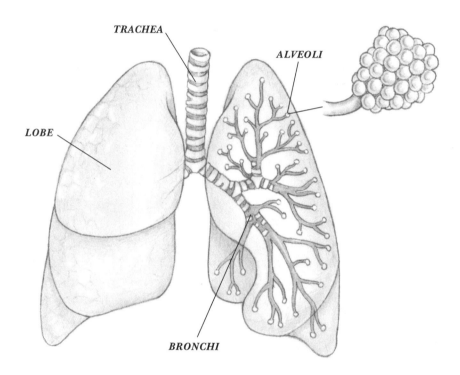

THE SPONGY TISSUE OF THE LUNGS ALLOWS THEM TO EXPAND AND FILL WITH OXYGEN AND CONTRACT TO EXPEL CARBON DIOXIDE. FRESH AIR FLOWS IN THROUGH THE WINDPIPE, OR TRACHEA, WHICH BRANCHES LIKE THE LIMBS OF A TREE TO FORM BRONCHI. THE BRONCHI TERMINATE IN AIR SACS, OR ALVEOLI, WHERE THE EXCHANGE OF OXYGEN AND WASTE—CARBON DIOXIDE—TAKES PLACE. WHILE THE OXYGEN ENTERS THE BLOODSTREAM, THE CARBON DIOXIDE MAKES THE REVERSE JOURNEY, AND EVENTUALLY IS EXHALED THROUGH THE TRACHEA. THE THREE SECTIONS OF THE RIGHT LUNG FILL THE CHEST, WHILE THE TWO SECTIONS OF THE LEFT LUNG LEAVE ROOM FOR THE HEART.

6. ARE YOU IN FREQUENT CONTACT WITH TOXIC SUBSTANCES AT WORK OR AT HOME? Repeated exposure to asbestos, radon, radiation, and environmental pollutants—particularly the by-products of diesel and other fossil fuels—can raise your lung cancer risk. Asbestos is especially hazardous to smokers.

7. DOES ANYONE IN YOUR FAMILY HAVE LUNG CANCER? Although lung cancer is not inherited, having a parent, sibling, or child with the disease more than doubles your risk. Some experts speculate that we inherit the ability—or inability—to metabolize toxic substances, which may affect our chances of developing lung cancer.

8. WERE YOU EVER TREATED FOR NON-HODGKIN'S LYMPHOMA OR HODGKIN'S DISEASE? Receiving radiation therapy for these cancers, especially at a young age, raises lung cancer risk.

9. HAVE YOU EVER HAD CANCER IN YOUR UPPER AIRWAY OR DIGESTIVE TRACT, PARTICULARLY CANCER OF THE LARYNX? People with a personal history of any of these diseases are more likely to develop lung cancer.

10. HAVE YOU EVER HAD LUNG CANCER BEFORE? The lifetime risk of a second primary cancer following early-stage lung cancer is 20 to 30 percent.

11. DO YOU HAVE A LUNG CONDITION SUCH AS CHRONIC OBSTRUCTIVE PULMONARY DISEASE, EMPHYSEMA, CHRONIC BRONCHITIS, OR TUBERCULOSIS? Any condition that obstructs the lungs, such as the scarring that follows tuberculosis, increases lung cancer risk.

CAUSES

Most lung cancers are non–small cell lung cancers. The group includes a subtype known as squamous cell carcinoma, which is most often associated with smoking.

Before cigarettes were factory-made and widely available, lung cancer was quite rare. Today tobacco is responsible for 80 to 90 percent of all lung cancer diagnoses and 87 percent of lung cancer deaths.

Inhaling tobacco smoke delivers large doses of toxic substances directly to the lungs. These toxic substances damage a host of genes—activating some, deactivating others, and interfering with those that direct cellular repair. The net effect of these genetic mutations is uncontrolled cell growth, the hallmark of cancer. Exposure to the by-products of tobacco smoke also increases the release of certain proteins called growth factors, which can contribute to the proliferation of abnormal cells. (As you'll see throughout part 2, smoking is a risk factor for many other cancers as well.)

And it isn't just cigarettes that are to blame. Smoking a pipe or cigar raises lung cancer risk, even if the smoke isn't inhaled. Exposure to secondhand cigar smoke at home or at work also elevates risk. Cigar smoke contains even more toxins than cigarette smoke, including irritants such as carbon monoxide, nicotine, and cyanide, as well as some 43 carcinogens such as nitrosamines, vinyl chloride, benzene, and arsenic.

Among other toxic substances associated with lung cancer, asbestos has been designated a group A carcinogen by the U.S. Environmental Protection Agency (EPA). It earned this dubious distinction after the EPA found convincing evidence that asbestos causes cancer in humans. Since 1989, when the EPA banned all new uses of asbestos, the prevalence of the substance in the environment has been on the decline. Still, it's a component of some 5,000 products, ranging from roofing and siding to wire insulation and brake linings.

Asbestos is a strong and flexible fiber, but it can break down to form a fine dust. When inhaled on a regular basis, this dust can cause cancer—particularly mesothelioma, which begins in the cells lining the outer surface of the lung. Asbestos exposure is second only to smoking as a cause of lung cancer.

Radon, another carcinogen with a connection to lung cancer, forms as uranium in the earth decays. Normally the radioactive gas—which is colorless, odorless, and tasteless—rises from the ground and dissipates into the atmosphere. But sometimes it accumulates in buildings, especially well-insulated ones from which it can't escape. When people in these buildings inhale the gas, it enters the bloodstream and circulates throughout the body. Over the course of this journey, the radon atoms decay. While some of the particles are exhaled into the environment, others linger in the lungs, where they can seriously damage the genetic material in the cells.

According to the EPA, "Radon in homes causes more deaths than fires, drowning, and airplane crashes combined." It is especially hazardous to children because they breathe faster than adults, and to pregnant women because the fetus gets a dose of radiation. Experts estimate that the incidence of lung cancer is about 10 times higher among those who are exposed to radon as teenagers than among those who first come into contact with the gas as 50-year-old adults.

The National Cancer Institute reports that the risk of lung cancer rises by 14 percent for a person who lives for 30 years in a house with a radon level of 4 picocuries per liter. That's the level at which the EPA recommends taking action. Breathing air with that concentration of the gas can deposit more than a half million radioactive particles in the lungs every hour. For comparison, the average radon level outdoors is 0.4 picocuries per liter.

Radon exposure is responsible for about 10 percent of all new lung cancer cases each year. An estimated one in four cases among nonsmokers may result from excessive radon levels in the home. According to the EPA, indoor radon is responsible for as many as 22,000 lung cancer deaths every year. And smoking raises the risk even more. In fact, smoking contributes to most radon-related deaths.

The conventional wisdom on air pollution was that it posed a greater risk for heart and lung conditions than for cancer per se. But a recent study challenged this widely accepted "fact" when it found a link between lung cancer and increased exposure to particulate matter in the air. The researchers associated fine particles and sulfur oxides with a higher death rate from several causes, including lung cancer. And according to another study, involving a half million adults in 100 cities, the risk of death from lung cancer rose in proportion to the concentration of fine particles in the air. One of the study's authors proposed that long-term exposure to air pollution may be as important a risk factor for lung cancer as is secondhand smoke.

SCREENING

A test that could detect lung cancer before it spreads and causes symptoms certainly would help reduce the number of deaths from the disease. But so far, none of the available diagnostic tools—such as chest x-ray and sputum cytology, which involves the examination of phlegm for abnormal cells—have caught a sufficient number of cancers early enough to be appropriate for routine use. Likewise, neither chest x-rays nor conventional CT scans have proven effective in reducing the chances of dying from lung cancer. But further research may provide the proof we need.

The 8-year National Lung Screening Trial now under way will compare chest x-rays and spiral computerized tomography (in which the scanning device rotates around the body rather than moving over it, as in a conventional CT scan) as tools for detecting early-stage lung cancer in smokers. Eventually, the trial will involve 50,000 current or former smokers at 30 medical centers throughout the United States. A spiral CT scan can detect a tumor less than 1 centimeter, or about ½ inch, in diameter, while a chest x-ray can spot a tumor twice that size. Usually, the smaller the tumor, the less advanced the cancer.

With the increasing availability of total-body scans at commercial sites, many people are opting to undergo this test, sometimes at their own expense. Experts disagree on the value of total-body scans for detecting lung cancer. One of the arguments is that because the scans don't distinguish between a harmless, benign nodule and cancer, a suspicious image may necessitate further, more invasive testing such as a lung biopsy to rule out cancer. These tests are costly and uncomfortable, and they can cause complications. What we need to determine is, are the costs of total-body scans and possible follow-up testing worth the benefits? And are these tests finding cancers early enough to warrant their general use? The results of the National Lung Screening Trial should help answer these questions.

Another large study—the Prostate, Lung, Colorectal, and Ovarian (PLCO) Screening Trial—is investigating the value of regular chest x-rays in detecting lung cancer and saving lives. The trial, which is sponsored by the National Cancer Institute, involves nearly 155,000 men and women between ages 55 and 74 in 10 cities across the United States. These volunteers will get chest x-rays at their initial visits, then once a year for 3 years. The researchers will track the study participants for 10 years.

If you are at high risk for lung cancer, according to the risk factors presented earlier in the chapter, you may want to consider enrolling in a clinical trial of screening tests like those described here. And if you develop any symptoms such as chest pain, cough, bloody sputum, or breathing problems, please consult your doctor right away—especially if you are a smoker. He may recommend a chest x-ray to take a closer look at your lungs.

PREVENTIVE STRATEGIES

Unlike many types of cancer, lung cancer is one in which the major risk factor—tobacco smoke—is avoidable. So if you're a smoker, quit. And if you're not, try to steer clear of situations that expose you to secondhand smoke.

Research at the Dana-Farber Cancer Institute in Boston shows that it's never too late to stop smoking. In a 10-year study, people who quit before starting treatment for lung cancer were less likely to die within 5 years than those who continued to smoke. Two years after therapy, only 16 percent of the smokers still were alive, compared with 28 percent of the former smokers.

The ease with which you can avoid secondhand smoke varies enormously depending on where you live. In California, for instance, legislators enacted the Law for a Smoke-Free Workplace to protect people from secondhand smoke in indoor work environments, including bars. Naturally, the legislation also had an impact on the people who frequent public places. Contrary to initial fears that restaurants and bars would lose business, their revenues actually increased during 1998, the first year after the law had passed. In one public opinion poll of bar patrons, two-thirds said that it was important for bars to be smoke-free. Other states range from having no smoking regulations (Georgia, North Carolina, and Idaho) to banning smoking in all workplaces and public buildings, including bars, restaurants, and casinos (New York and Delaware).

If your workplace is not smoke-free and you are in a position to institute change, *Making Your Workplace Smokefree: A Decision Maker's Guide* (a booklet from the Centers for Disease Control and Prevention Office on Smoking and Health) offers sound advice for creating a no-smoking policy. Even if you're not in that position, you may want to raise the issue with your supervisor or someone on your company's human resources staff.

But don't simply wait for change to come. You can be proactive about protecting your own body. For instance, if one of your coworkers is a smoker, discreetly ask the person to light up outside because you're concerned about how the secondhand smoke will affect your health.

At home, of course, you're in charge. You can ask guests to refrain from smoking. Even better, put away any ashtrays before they arrive.

Testing your home for radon is important if you live in an area that has uranium in the soil. Just keep in mind that even though radon levels are higher in some locations than in others, so-called hot spots can occur anywhere, according to the EPA. Radon test kits are available at most home improvement and hardware stores. For more information, call the EPA's radon hot line at (800) SOS-RADON, or visit its Web site at www.epa.gov/iaq/radon.

Keep in mind that exposure to radon or tobacco smoke does not guarantee that you will get lung cancer. You can minimize their impact by taking steps to control other cancer risk factors. And the best place to start is with your diet.

We know, for example, that people who have been exposed to tobacco smoke are more likely to develop lung cancer if they eat few or no fruits and vegetables. Conversely, many large-scale studies have shown that eating foods rich in antioxidants, especially beta-carotene, reduces lung cancer risk.

Fruits seem to be especially protective. In a European study of male smokers, the more fruit the heavy smokers ate, the less chance they had of developing lung cancer. Another study found that eating lots of apples significantly reduced cancer risk, probably because apples are rich in plant compounds (phytochemicals) called flavonoids. Other sources of flavonoids include cruciferous vegetables, such as broccoli, cabbage, and Brussels sprouts. They, too, protect against lung cancer.

CHEMOPREVENTION

While studies to explore the preventive benefits of antioxidant-rich foods have produced impressive results, the same cannot be said for research that attempted to zero in on the specific micronutrients responsible for the protective effects. Neither beta-carotene alone nor a beta-carotene/vitamin E combination prevented lung cancer. In fact, two of three large studies—the Alpha Tocopherol Beta Carotene Study and the Carotene and Retinol Efficacy Trial—found that large doses of beta-carotene increased the incidence of lung cancer in people who smoked and in those exposed to asbestos. In the Physicians' Health Study, beta-carotene had no effect on lung cancer risk in current or former smokers. (There's no evidence that beta-carotene raises lung cancer risk in nonsmokers.)

The lesson from these studies, combined with epidemiological research, is that a whole food is more likely than a specific micronutrient to protect against cancer. It may be that a certain combination of nutrients in a food, or another as yet unidentified component of a food, is responsible for the reduction in cancer risk. Or it may be that people exposed to tobacco smoke respond to the by-products of beta-carotene metabolism differently than others do.

What we do know is that antioxidant supplements—and perhaps high-dose ones in particular—do not have the same effect on the body and the cancer process as whole foods do. For this reason, while we recommend eating fruits and vegetables and taking a daily multivitamin, we advise against shoring up your antioxidant intake with supplements.

At least two clinical trials currently under way are attempting to determine whether certain drugs can reverse precancerous conditions and prevent lung cancer in former smokers. One of these trials is investigating celecoxib, which blocks the COX-2 enzyme that is associated with the growth of cancer cells. The other is using an asthma drug, zileuton, to see if it can reverse abnormal changes in lung cells. This trial includes former smokers who have not developed cancer, as well as people who have been treated for early-stage lung cancer or head and neck cancers.

WHAT YOU CAN DO NOW TO PREVENT LUNG CANCER

1. If you smoke, quit.

2. If you live with a smoker, talk with the person about the health implications of his or her secondhand smoke. Do what you can to help the person kick the habit. If the person insists on lighting up, ask him or her not to smoke in the house or in the car.

3. If your workplace permits smoking, talk with your coworkers who smoke about the hazards of their habit to them and to you. Ask them to go outside when they light up. Be proactive about lobbying for a smoke-free workplace.

4. Steer clear of restaurants, bars, and other public establishments that allow smoking.

5. Eat at least five, and preferably nine, servings of fruits and vegetables every day. If you are a current or former smoker, be especially generous with your fruit consumption. And get plenty of yellow/orange vegetables, which are rich in beta-carotene and other carotenoids.

6. Test your home for radon, especially if you live in an area that has high radon levels or is a known "hot spot."

7. If you are at high risk for lung cancer—for instance, you're a smoker and you've been exposed to asbestos—consider enrolling in a clinical trial of screening tests.

CHAPTER 11

COLORECTAL

CANCER

· · · · · · · ·

FOR 2004, EXPERTS PROJECT that colorectal cancer—that is, cancer of the colon or rectum—will affect some 146,940 Americans. No wonder it currently ranks as the third most common cancer among both men and women in the United States. In fact, as many as 6 percent of Americans will develop colorectal cancer sometime in their lives.

Now for the good news: We know for certain that by removing precancerous growths called polyps, or adenomas, we actually can prevent invasive colorectal cancer. Proof comes from research like the National Polyp Study, which found that the incidence of colorectal cancer was 75 percent lower among people who had undergone surgery to remove intestinal polyps than among those who hadn't.

Increases in screening and in treating intestinal polyps probably helped to reduce the incidence of colorectal cancer by 1.8 percent a year in the late 1980s and early 1990s. Since then, the incidence has remained stable. The mortality rate for colorectal cancer—the number of people who die from the disease—has declined as well. While colorectal cancer still accounts for about 10 percent of all cancer deaths, the number of deaths has dropped by 1.7 percent a year for the past 15 years.

Unfortunately, colorectal cancer remains an even more serious health concern for African-Americans. Compared with other ethnic groups, they have the highest incidence of the disease, with as many as 45.2 women per 100,000 and 58.3 men per 100,000 getting diagnosed every year. African-American women are more likely to die from colorectal cancer than women in other racial groups, with a death rate of 19.9 per 100,000. Among African-American men, the death rate is 27.7 per 100,000—the highest of both genders and all ethnic groups.

ARE YOU AT RISK?

1. ARE YOU OVER AGE 40? For both men and women, the risk of colorectal cancer begins rising after 40, with a sharp increase in the early fifties. Then risk doubles with each subsequent decade.

2. ARE YOU OF ASHKENAZI JEWISH DESCENT? Estimates are that about 6 percent of Ashkenazi Jews inherit a genetic mutation that increases the risk of colorectal cancer.

3. DO YOU HAVE A FAMILY HISTORY OF COLORECTAL CANCER OR INTESTINAL POLYPS? While three in four people who develop colorectal cancer have no family history of it, a 45-year-old who does has three times the average risk of developing the disease.

4. DO YOU HAVE A FAMILY HISTORY OF A HEREDITARY COLORECTAL CANCER SYNDROME? People who inherit the gene mutations for hereditary nonpolyposis colon cancer (HNPCC) have a 70 percent lifetime risk of developing colorectal cancer. Among those who inherit familial adenomatous polyposis (FAP), 100 percent will develop colorectal cancer by the time they turn 40 unless they pursue medical intervention, usually surgical removal of the colon.

5. DO YOU HAVE A PERSONAL HISTORY OF INTESTINAL POLYPS? Cancer is present in about 5 percent of polyps.

6. DO YOU HAVE A PERSONAL HISTORY OF CHRONIC INFLAMMATORY BOWEL DISEASE (ULCERATIVE COLITIS

OR CROHN'S DISEASE)? Anyone who has a medical problem that causes the intestine to become inflamed for a long period of time is 30 times more likely to develop colorectal cancer than someone who's healthy. Some of these inflammatory disorders, like Crohn's, tend to run in families.

The Large Intestine

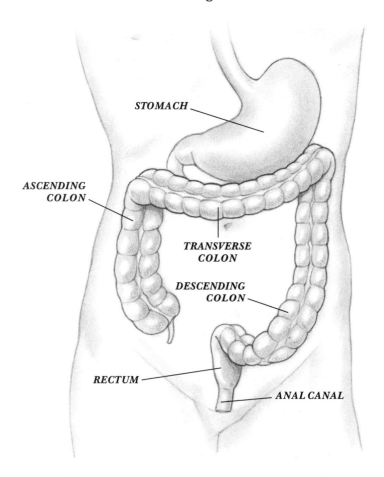

THE MAIN FUNCTIONS OF THE LARGE INTESTINE, OR COLON, ARE TO ABSORB WATER AND TRANSPORT WASTE. WASTE PASSES THROUGH IT ON ITS WAY TO THE RECTUM AND ANAL CANAL, WHERE IT EXITS THE BODY. FROM END TO END, THE LARGE INTESTINE IS ABOUT 6 FEET LONG.

7. DO YOU SMOKE? In 1997, experts estimated that as many as 12 percent of colorectal cancer deaths in the United States could be attributed to smoking. According to the American Cancer Society's Cancer Prevention Study II, female smokers were at least 40 percent more likely to die from colorectal cancer than women who never had lit up. Male smokers were 30 percent more likely to die from the disease.

8. DO YOU DRINK ALCOHOL? People who do, particularly men who drink beer, are at increased risk for colorectal cancer.

9. ARE YOU SEDENTARY? We don't know for certain whether physical inactivity itself is a risk factor for colorectal cancer, or if it's implicated in the disease because of its association with other risk factors, such as genetic predisposition or diet. For example, the link between a diet high in saturated fat and colorectal cancer is stronger in people who are sedentary than in those who are active.

10. DOES YOUR USUAL DIET CONTAIN A LOT OF FAT, ESPECIALLY FROM ANIMAL SOURCES, AND/OR LITTLE FIBER, WITH FEW FRUITS AND VEGETABLES? Studies that have tracked large groups of people to establish a link between fat or meat consumption and colorectal cancer have produced mixed results. But we do know that the incidence of the disease is higher in countries where people get nearly half their daily calories from fat, compared with countries where fat accounts for only 10 percent of a typical day's calorie intake. Some studies indicate that fiber could help protect against colorectal cancer.

11. ARE YOU OBESE? Men who are obese are 40 percent more likely to develop colorectal cancer than men who maintain a healthy weight. Both men and women may be more likely to die from this cancer if they are overweight.

CAUSES

Colorectal cancer is one of the few cancers that are largely preventable because we can find and remove precancerous growths before they turn malignant. Tests to detect early-stage cancer, which is highly treatable, also are widely available.

But just what causes polyps to form in the first place, and what causes about 5 percent of these growths to become malignant, is not completely understood. Except for inherited forms of the disease, which result from a specific genetic mutation, colorectal cancer appears to arise from the combination of genetic mutations and environmental factors such as poor diet or exposure to carcinogens in the intestine.

COLORECTAL CANCER GENES

About 16 percent of all colorectal cancer cases are inherited. Scientists have identified several genes that can make a person highly susceptible to the disease.

For example, an inherited mutation in the adenomatous polyposis coli (APC) gene, which normally slows cell growth, causes a rare condition in which hundreds of polyps form in the intestine, usually by the time the person is a teenager. If untreated, the condition—familial adenomatous polyposis—inevitably leads to colorectal cancer. In fact, about 1 percent of the colorectal cancer cases diagnosed each year result from familial adenomatous polyposis (FAP). A similar inherited condition, called Gardner syndrome, also causes polyps to form in the intestine.

Another genetic mutation, this one affecting as many as six different genes that direct DNA repair, allows polyps to grow unusually fast. This sets the stage for hereditary nonpolyposis colon cancer, which accounts for about 3 percent of all colorectal cancer cases.

Colorectal cancer does tend to run in families even in the absence of a specific genetic disorder or an inherited pattern to the disease. By the same token, the gene mutation that causes FAP appears in some noninherited colorectal cancers, too.

DIET

The incidence of colorectal cancer varies tremendously throughout different parts of the world. This has led researchers to suspect that some dietary factor may be responsible for the larger number of cancer cases in the United States, northern Europe, and Australia, compared with Asia, Africa, and parts of Latin America. We do know that people who move from a country of low risk to one of high risk are more likely to develop colorectal cancer than those who stay behind.

Even within the same country, colorectal cancer risk rises as dietary habits change. This was seen in Japan, where deaths from colorectal cancer more than doubled over a 30-year period—from 1955 to 1985—during which the traditional diet and lifestyle gave way to modern influences.

The most obvious difference between countries with a low risk of colorectal cancer and those with a high risk is the amount of fat and fiber in their respective diets. Yet oddly enough, research efforts to identify and substantiate a direct link between dietary fat, fiber, and colorectal cancer have produced mixed results. The same is true for the amounts of fruits and vegetables in various diets: While people who live in countries with a low risk of colorectal cancer tend to eat more of these foods, researchers have not been able to conclusively establish a protective effect.

Both fat intake and calorie intake indirectly contribute to colorectal cancer by causing obesity. People who weigh more than they should produce excessive amounts of chemicals called growth factors, particularly insulin-like growth factor-1 (IGF-1). This chemical stimulates the growth of premalignant and malignant cells as well as healthy ones.

Dietary fat also may contribute to colorectal cancer by triggering the secretion of larger-than-normal amounts of bile acid from the gallbladder into the intestine. Just how this might influence the cancer process isn't known. Research has shown that calcium may help reduce the risk of colorectal cancer by binding with bile acid. We also know that adults who consume about 700 milligrams of calcium a day are 40 to 50 percent less likely than average to develop colorectal cancer. What remains unclear is which form of calcium is best and whether calcium from dairy products is more effective than supplements.

Many experts believe that the higher rate of colorectal cancer in Western countries may have something to do with the amount of red meat in their traditional diets. Here especially, fat and calories may come into play, since most cuts of red meat contain ample amounts of both. But cooking method also is a factor. When meat is subjected to high temperatures during frying, boiling, or barbecuing, the juices burn, which leads to the formation of cancer-causing compounds called heterocyclic amines.

We suspect that colorectal cancer risk most likely is under the influence of more than just one or two dietary factors, which may help explain why studies that single out individual factors for testing have not shown a conclusive link. Another possible reason for the lack of clear evidence on the relationship between diet and colorectal cancer is that consuming certain food components, such as fiber, shows a significant benefit only after many, many years.

In fact, the American Gastroenterological Association points out in its guidelines that it's important not only to eat more fiber but also to start sooner rather than later—at least 10 to 20 years before the age at which the incidence of colorectal cancer peaks. A reduction in risk probably results from the combination of lots of fiber, less fat and modest calories, and at least five servings of fruits and vegetables a day.

LIFESTYLE HABITS

Many studies have established a connection between drinking alcohol and smoking and a rise in colorectal cancer risk. The theory is that alcohol stimulates cell growth within the mucous lining of the intestine and possibly allows carcinogens to travel to the farthest reaches of the large intestine. With smoking, the poor eating habits typical among those who light up may be to blame.

As mentioned earlier, we still aren't sure how a sedentary lifestyle might contribute to colorectal cancer. We do know that a person who doesn't engage in regular exercise misses out on benefits like maintaining a healthy weight and improving the movement of waste through the intestinal tract—both of which may help protect against colorectal cancer.

On a related note, bowel habits may influence colorectal cancer risk if a person doesn't move his or her bowels on a regular basis. This allows carcinogens in the waste to remain in contact with the walls of the intestine for a prolonged period of time. In general, people who drink lots of water and eat healthy amounts of fiber from a variety of sources, including fruits and vegetables, don't have problems with constipation. If they also limit their fat intakes, their stools will remain soft and pass easily.

SCREENING

Although screening tests for colorectal cancer are widely available, only half of all adults age 50 and older have ever had a fecal occult blood test, and only one-third have had a sigmoidoscopy or colonoscopy within the past 5 years. One reason is that despite the American Cancer Society screening guidelines, many health care providers don't routinely advise their patients to get these screening tests. And when they do, their patients may not be comfortable with the procedures or the preparation beforehand, and so don't readily follow the doctors' orders. Of course, some people don't get regular colorectal cancer screenings because either they lack health insurance or their insurers won't cover the costs.

Currently, the American Cancer Society recommends one of the following screening options for men and women age 50 and older who are at average risk for colorectal cancer:

- Fecal occult blood test every year
- Flexible sigmoidoscopy every 5 years
- Colonoscopy every 10 years
- Double-contrast barium enema every 5 years

Anyone with a personal history of colorectal cancer, a strong family history of colorectal cancer or intestinal polyps, a personal history of chronic inflammatory bowel disease, or a family history of hereditary colorectal cancer syndromes should discuss earlier and/or more frequent screening with their physicians. With these guidelines in mind, let's look at each screening test in turn.

FECAL OCCULT BLOOD TEST

The word *occult* means "hidden." So as its name suggests, this test detects blood in the feces that is not visible to the naked eye. Blood in the stool may be a sign of colorectal cancer, though it also can indicate several other medical problems. Intestinal polyps, for example, may bleed as waste passes by them, rupturing their fragile blood vessels. Hemorrhoids, which actually are enlarged veins, can cause blood in the stool. So, too, can diverticulosis, an inflammation of the colon that is very common among people middle-aged and older.

For these reasons, it's important to remember that a positive fecal occult blood test indicates only the presence of blood in the stool. It doesn't give a clue as to why the blood is there, so further investigation is necessary.

By the same token, a negative test result—that is, no blood in the stool—doesn't mean that a person is cancer-free. Not all colorectal cancers bleed, nor do they bleed continuously. The fecal occult blood test may miss cancers that are not causing symptoms. This is why a sigmoidoscopy every 5 years or a colonoscopy every 10 years also is a good idea, regardless of the fecal occult results.

You can perform the fecal occult blood test on your own at home, with a test kit from your doctor or the drugstore. Typically, the kit involves using a small wooden stick to smear a sample of fecal material on a test card, which you then must mail to a laboratory for analysis. Stool from the toilet paper also can be put on the card. You will need to collect samples from three separate bowel movements. Space for the three samples may be on one card or on three separate cards.

Before starting the test, be sure to read the directions carefully. For instance, you may be instructed not to take aspirin, ibuprofen, or certain other pain medications for a week prior to testing because they can cause minor bleeding. Likewise, eating red meat within 3 days of the test can contribute to a false positive result. A similar outcome may occur when taking vitamin C or eating radishes, turnips, horseradish, or melon within 3 days of testing, as they contain a chemical that can alter the results.

Some newer tests, known as immunochemical tests, rely on laboratory-made antibodies to detect a substance in red blood cells in the stool. Since the antibodies don't react with food or nutrients, they are less likely to give an inaccurate reading. They also are easier to use. One immunochemical test already approved in the United States involves swiping a long-handled brush over the surface of the stool in the toilet bowl and then dabbing a sample onto a test card. When the card dries, you mail it to the laboratory.

No matter which type of fecal occult blood test you choose, be sure to call your doctor for the results. You may not get them otherwise.

SIGMOIDOSCOPY

The sigmoidoscope is a flexible, tubelike instrument that allows a physician to inspect the left side of the bowel—the lowest portion—for any abnormalities, including polyps. If he notices anything suspicious, he can take a photo with a tiny camera at the end of the sigmoidoscope. He also can use the instrument to remove a sample of tissue for further examination.

Prior to a sigmoidoscopy, you'll need to cleanse your bowel as much as possible by consuming only clear liquids for dinner the night before. Your doctor may recommend taking a laxative, and possibly an enema or two, as part of the preparation process.

For the actual test, your doctor will thoroughly lubricate the sigmoidoscope before gently inserting it through the rectum and into the colon for a distance of about 2 feet. You may feel some cramping during the examination, which lasts 10 to 20 minutes, but you shouldn't need any pain medication. Your doctor may offer a sedative such as Valium so you can relax during the procedure.

COLONOSCOPY

Much like the sigmoidoscope, the colonoscope is a flexible, tubelike instrument with a light and a microscopic video camera at the end—only the colonoscope is long enough that it can inspect the entire colon at once. The instrument also allows for the extraction of tissue samples for analysis, as well as for the removal of any polyps that may turn up during the procedure.

Because the colonoscope runs the full length of the large intestine, a colonoscopy can be painful. For this reason, your doctor likely will recommend sedation for the 30- to 40-minute examination. He also will provide instructions for an extensive preparation process, again because you must empty the entire large intestine. In general, you may have only clear liquids the day before the test, along with a special fluid or laxative—or both—to flush out your intestines. An enema or two can help ensure that the bowel is completely empty.

DOUBLE-CONTRAST BARIUM ENEMA

Before colonoscopy and sigmoidoscopy became so widely available, the double-contrast barium enema was the most common procedure for visually inspecting the colon. It involves filling the colon with barium and air so polyps will stand out on an x-ray.

The preparation for the double-contrast barium enema is similar to those for the other screening tests. For 1 to 3 days prior to testing, you can eat only liquids, and no dairy products. You cannot have anything by mouth after midnight the night before the test. In the morning, you may need to take a laxative or an enema to be sure that you've emptied your colon of all waste.

Once you're in the x-ray room, you'll be given an enema with barium. The barium and air remain in your bowels for the x-rays. In fact, you may be asked to turn several times so the barium fills your entire colon. You can empty your bowels as soon as the x-rays are complete.

While this test is uncomfortable because of the urge to have a bowel movement, it generally isn't painful. Nevertheless, doctors rarely use it as a screening technique. The American Cancer Society still includes the double-contrast barium enema in its guidelines because in certain situations—for example, at hospitals in rural areas—the test may be the only one available to check for polyps. If it happens that a polyp is found during the test, another procedure is necessary to remove the growth.

TESTS IN DEVELOPMENT

Advances in medical technology have led to significant improvements in screening tests for colorectal cancer. Researchers are studying whether the following tests might be as effective for detecting early-stage cancers and precancerous growths as those already available.

VIRTUAL COLONOSCOPY. This test, which also goes by the name CT colonography, uses computer-assisted tomography (CT scanning) to create 2-D and/or 3-D images of the entire colon. The 10-minute test offers many benefits, but further clinical study is required to determine if virtual colonoscopy is as good as conventional colonoscopy at detecting polyps and if any improvement in accuracy is worth the potentially higher cost for the test.

So far, virtual colonoscopy appears as effective as conventional colonoscopy in spotting large polyps. This may be enough, since polyps grow slowly and cancer more likely will be present in larger growths. In addition, virtual colonoscopy may be better than the conventional test at finding cancers where the intestine forms thick folds. Some studies suggest that virtual colonoscopy is 100 percent effective in detecting cancers.

But virtual colonoscopy isn't as simple as the word *virtual* may imply. People get the mistaken impression that since it doesn't involve inserting some sort of scope into the colon, the test is as effortless as having an x-ray. Virtual colonoscopy still requires bowel cleansing beforehand. It also involves pumping air or carbon dioxide through the rectum into the colon, using a thin probe about the size of a rectal thermometer. The air or gas expands the folds in the colon walls so any polyps that may be hiding there become visible. This part of the test is somewhat uncomfortable—some say as uncomfortable as conventional colonoscopy—but it usually isn't painful.

During the CT scan, you will be asked to turn over so the radiologist can collect images while you're faceup and facedown. Afterward, you may experience some cramping. But since the procedure doesn't require sedation, you should be able to resume your usual activities right away.

Virtual colonoscopy offers more advantages than just speed and no sedation. The radiologist can manipulate the images to show the colon walls from various perspectives. In effect, the images simulate what would be seen with conventional colonoscopy (hence the name virtual colonoscopy). As with the instant photos and videos obtained through a colonoscope, the images from the CT scan can be saved to compare with others in the future.

One disadvantage of virtual colonoscopy: If the test happens to find a suspicious growth, a follow-up procedure—most likely conventional colonoscopy—will be necessary to remove it.

MOLECULAR STOOL TESTING. Colorectal cancer cells contain many genetic mutations that create a kind of biological signature for distinguishing their DNA from the DNA of normal cells. By looking for certain "hot spots," or specific changes in the DNA of cells that pass in the feces, doctors could detect a malignancy before it causes symptoms. To date, the most studied molecular stool test is PreGen-26, manufactured by EXACT Sciences Corporation.

While molecular stool testing still is under evaluation, it seems most suitable as an adjunct to conventional colonoscopy, rather than as a replacement for it. On the other hand, it may prove more reliable than the fecal occult blood test. This is because cells from any abnormal growth in the intestine shed continuously and abundantly into the stool, even if the growths themselves don't bleed. In a study comparing molecular stool testing and fecal occult blood testing, the former detected 8 of 11 advanced benign growths, compared with none for the latter.

Molecular stool testing also has an advantage over sigmoidoscopy. Viewing the lower portion of the colon with a sigmoidoscope detects polyps or cancers only in that area. But a positive result on a molecular stool test indicates the presence of an abnormality anywhere along the large intestine. In an early study comparing the two screening tests, molecular stool testing identified DNA changes in 97 of 110 cancers that examination with a sigmoidoscope had missed.

Because molecular stool testing doesn't present the inconvenience, risk, or discomfort of other colorectal cancer screening tests, people may be more willing to undergo the procedure. Right now, it is rather expensive—about $400 per test. But eventually it may be automated, which will help rein in the cost. For these reasons, we suspect that molecular stool testing may become the screening tool of choice for colorectal cancer and precancers.

Thus far, studies indicate that molecular stool testing can detect about 50 percent of colorectal cancers. We think that it may be most helpful as a periodic screening test when a routine colonoscopy produces normal results, especially in those at high risk.

CAPSULE VIDEO ENDOSCOPY. TV and newspaper reporters have described this new technology as a "camera in a capsule." That's exactly what the M2A capsule is. A miniaturized camera snaps images second by second as it makes an 8-hour journey through the digestive tract. Then a computer creates a video from the images.

Unlike any of the screening tests described so far, the M2A capsule can spot abnormalities in the small intestine, not just the large intestine or colon. Despite the appeal of this technology, it has its shortcomings—such as the possibility of missing suspicious areas not in the camera's view. These and other problems need to be overcome before capsule video endoscopy becomes widely available as a screening or diagnostic test for colorectal cancer.

PREVENTIVE STRATEGIES

Despite the mixed results of studies examining the relationship between diet and colorectal cancer, research involving large groups of people has found a lower incidence of colorectal cancer among those who get lots of fiber from a variety of sources, including an abundance of fruits and vegetables. These observations are too impressive to dismiss. We also have seen increases in colorectal cancer risk with too many calories; too much fat, meat (red and white), and alcohol; and too little calcium and possibly folate. Though just how these dietary factors might contribute to the cancer process remains unclear, we agree with the American Cancer Society's recommendation to follow a low-fat, high-fiber diet.

With regard to fiber, the American Gastroenterological Association offers a more specific recommendation: between 30 and 35 grams a day, which is about three times the Recommended Dietary Allowance. This fiber should come from a variety of sources, including fruits, vegetables, legumes, and whole grains. Eating more fiber is a good idea for a number of reasons beyond protecting against colorectal cancer—such as lowering cholesterol and blood pressure, improving the body's response to insulin, and preventing coronary artery disease.

Since running low on calcium or folate may raise the risk of colon cancer, we recommend getting a total of 1,500 milligrams of calcium and 400 micrograms of folate every day. Most multivitamins contain folate (or folic acid), but you probably will need to take calcium as a separate supplement to make sure that you're getting enough.

The research evidence of an association between excessive alcohol consumption and colorectal cancer ranges from weak to strong. Still, we recommend that men limit themselves to two drinks a day, and women to one drink a day. A drink equals 12 ounces of regular beer, 5 ounces of wine, or a cocktail made with 1½ ounces of 80-proof distilled spirits.

Quitting smoking is one of the most important measures for protecting against various forms of cancer, including colorectal cancer. People who smoke a pack a day are 50 percent more likely to develop colorectal cancer than those who never have smoked. The good news that your risk will decline every year once you quit.

Some research shows that an active lifestyle can reduce colorectal cancer risk by as much as 40 to 50 percent. What isn't clear is whether the reduction results from the activity itself or from other healthy habits that usually accompany an active lifestyle, such as a nutritious diet. Still, increasing your activity level is wise for improving your overall health and lowering your risk of numerous chronic diseases, including cancer. The American Cancer Society recommends at least 30 minutes of physical activity at least 5 days a week—though 45 minutes of moderate to vigorous activity is even better.

If you have a family history of colorectal cancer, you may want to discuss genetic testing with your doctor or a genetic counselor. Tests are available to identify the gene mutations associated with familial adenomatous polyposis and hereditary nonpolyposis colon cancer. Some people with FAP, which almost inevitably leads to cancer, choose to have surgery to remove their colons—often while still in their early twenties. This procedure usually isn't recommended for those with HNPCC, which carries a lower risk of colorectal cancer than FAP.

CHEMOPREVENTION

In December 1999, the U.S. Food and Drug Administration approved the COX-2 inhibitor celecoxib (Celebrex) as a treatment for people with FAP. The hope is that celexocib, which doesn't appear to irritate the stomach as other nonsteroidal anti-inflammatory drugs can, will delay the need for polyp removal until the teen years or later. In one study involving 80 people, published the year after celexocib received approval for this purpose, those who took 400 milligrams of Celebrex twice a day showed a 30 percent reduction in polyps, compared with those who took either 100 milligrams or a placebo.

Because other studies have shown that people who take aspirin and NSAIDs are 50 percent less likely to develop intestinal polyps and colorectal cancer, clinical trials are under way to assess the protective effects of these drugs. It could be that people who already are taking a baby aspirin a day to reduce their risk of heart attack or stroke may be lowering their risk of colorectal cancer as well. But until further research proves its benefit, we don't recommend a daily low-dose aspirin for everyone. Those with inherited conditions that place them at high risk for colorectal cancer should discuss this preventive measure with their physicians.

Hormone replacement therapy appears to slightly lower colorectal cancer risk. For postmenopausal women who are at high risk for the disease, it's another factor to discuss with their gynecologists when weighing the pros and cons of HRT for relief from menopausal discomforts.

Several trials currently in progress are exploring whether and how various chemopreventives might interrupt the colorectal cancer process. One active area of research involves various dosages of curcumin, a component of the spice turmeric. An antioxidant, curcumin may inhibit the COX-2 enzyme much like celecoxib.

Meanwhile, researchers at three cancer centers—two in the United States and one in Great Britain—are comparing celecoxib alone with the combination of celecoxib and difluoromethylornithine (DFMO), a drug that prevents cells from reproducing. Another study is examining the protective effects of DFMO and the COX-2 inhibitor sulindac in volunteers who already have undergone polyp removal. Furthest along is a clinical trial of the drug exisulind to prevent polyps in people with familial adenomatous polyposis.

Eventually, researchers may conclude that more than one preventive measure is necessary to lower the risk of colorectal cancer. This is why a number of studies are looking into the safety and effectiveness of various combinations, like increasing intakes of fiber and calcium while taking drugs such as DFMO and sulindac. At this time, no chemopreventive is recommended for people with an average risk of colorectal cancer.

WHAT YOU CAN DO NOW
TO PREVENT COLORECTAL CANCER

1. Follow the American Cancer Society screening guidelines that are appropriate for your age and colorectal cancer risk.

2. Aim for at least five, and preferably nine, servings of fruits and vegetables every day.

3. Consume 30 to 35 grams of fiber a day from a variety of sources.

4. Limit your intake of dietary fat to no more than 30 percent of your total daily calories.

5. Engage in at least 30 minutes of moderate physical activity at least 5 days a week, and try to work up to at least 45 minutes of moderate to vigorous activity at least 5 days a week.

6. Maintain a healthy weight. (For help in determining just what is healthy for you, see page 225.)

7. If you smoke, quit.

8. If you drink, limit yourself to two alcoholic beverages a day if you're a man, one if you're a woman.

9. Take 1,500 milligrams of calcium and 400 micrograms of folate (folic acid) a day.

10. If you are at high risk for colorectal cancer, talk with your doctor about taking a low dose of aspirin or an NSAID every day as a preventive measure.

CHAPTER 12

OVARIAN

CANCER

• • • • • • •

OVARIAN CANCER—WHICH CAN AFFECT either of a woman's two ovaries—has been on the decline over the past decade. While the incidence is low, it remains the sixth most common cancer among women, accounting for about 4 percent of all cancer cases and affecting an estimated 25,580 women in 2004. It also is the most lethal.

Part of the reason is that early detection of ovarian cancer is very difficult. Symptoms of a small tumor can be vague and may not point directly to a problem in the ovaries. For example, digestive problems (such as abdominal bloating, indigestion, and gas), pelvic or lower back pain, and frequent urination also occur with many other, less serious conditions. When ovarian cancer is caught at an early stage, often it's because a tumor turns up by chance during surgery for something else.

More than half of all women with ovarian cancer are in an advanced stage of the disease by the time they find out what's wrong. At that point, their prognosis is poor. Today ovarian cancer is the fifth leading cause of cancer deaths in women, and the leading cause of death among cancers of the female reproductive organs.

Still, ovarian cancer is not a common malignancy. In the United States, a woman has about a 2 percent chance of developing the disease sometime in her life.

ARE YOU AT RISK?

1. ARE YOU MIDDLE-AGED OR OLDER? Like most cancers, ovarian cancer tends occur later in life. The average age at diagnosis for epithelial ovarian cancer, the most common form of the disease, is about 59.

2. DOES YOUR MOTHER, SISTER, OR DAUGHTER HAVE OVARIAN CANCER? Although most women who develop ovarian cancer do not have a family history of the disease, someone who inherited a genetic predisposition from her mother or father has nearly a 1-in-10 chance of getting it. If a woman's mother, sister, or daughter has ovarian cancer, her own risk is about 5 percent. It bumps up to 7 percent if two or more first-degree relatives have the disease.

3. ARE YOU OF ASHKENAZI JEWISH DESCENT? About 39 percent of ovarian cancers in Ashkenazi Jewish women are associated with mutations in the BRCA1 or BRCA2 gene. Women who carry either or both of these mutations have a 16.5 percent lifetime risk of developing ovarian cancer.

4. DOES ANY MEMBER OF YOUR FAMILY—MALE OR FEMALE—CARRY A MUTATED BRCA1 OR BRCA2 GENE, AS DETERMINED THROUGH GENETIC TESTING? If so, you have a 50 percent chance of carrying the mutation, too. In that case, you may want to consider genetic testing for yourself.

5. HAVE YOU HAD BREAST CANCER? Women who develop breast cancer at an early age or who have a family history of the disease—or both—are at especially high risk for ovarian cancer and may have inherited mutated BRCA genes. According to a Swedish study of more than 30,000 women, those who were under age 40 when they received their breast cancer diagnoses were three times as likely to develop ovarian cancer as those who were older at diagnosis. The disease risk was four times higher for women with family histories of breast and ovarian cancers among first-degree female relatives. And those with both risk factors—early diagnosis and family history—were 17 times as likely to develop ovarian cancer as women who didn't have breast cancer.

6. DO YOU HAVE HEREDITARY NONPOLYPOSIS CO-LORECTAL CANCER? Having this type of cancer raises your risk of ovarian and endometrial cancers.

7. DO YOU HAVE A LONG HISTORY OF UNINTER-RUPTED OVULATION? If you began menstruating before age 12, have never been pregnant or first gave birth after age 30, and/or went through menopause after age 50, you've had many years of uninterrupted ovulation. This appears to increase ovarian cancer risk.

QUESTIONABLE RISKS

You may have heard about a possible link between fertility drugs—that is, drugs that stimulate ovulation—and ovarian cancer. So far, the findings of research to confirm this link have been inconsistent. It's true that in some studies, women who failed to become pregnant when taking fertility drugs were more likely to develop ovarian cancer. But the risk may stem from the infertility itself rather than from the drugs that treat it. In fact, research involving women who did become pregnant after treatment showed little increased risk.

One theory proposes that infertility or difficulty becoming pregnant itself is a risk factor for ovarian cancer, and the use of a fertility drug is simply a marker for that risk. Another maintains that long-term use of these drugs is the problem. One study did show that women who had taken fertility drugs for longer than a year were more likely to develop tumors, though in general the growths were of a type with a low potential for malignancy.

Until we have more definitive information about the link between fertility drugs and ovarian cancer, women who are struggling to become pregnant should work with their doctors to determine whether they should take ovulation-stimulating drugs. After all, ovarian cancer is a theoretical risk that must be weighed against the immediate reality of a woman's desire to become pregnant. Fertility drugs are a reasonable choice if pregnancy is a priority. But we do recommend limiting treatment to no more than six cycles.

Another unproven risk factor is the use of talc-containing body powder. Researchers found a slightly higher risk of ovarian cancer in women who applied talc to the genital area. This may be due to the fact that more than 20 years ago, talcum powder sometimes contained asbestos, a known carcinogen. Today it's illegal for talc to contain asbestos, and asbestos-free powders have no substantiated link to ovarian cancer. Nevertheless, we do advise our patients to avoid so-called feminine hygiene products. The vagina is not a dirty place, so there is no need to put powder on the genitals or to douche. A daily shower or bath is adequate.

Occasionally we see health warnings circulating via e-mail about the dangers of tampons. Some of these Internet rumors say that the asbestos in tampons is harmful; others claim that a chemical used to bleach the

The Ovaries

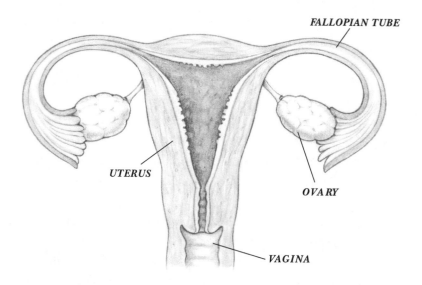

THE TWO ALMOND-SHAPED OVARIES SIT TO EITHER SIDE OF THE UTERUS, JUST BELOW THE FALLOPIAN TUBES. EACH MONTH ONE OF THE OVARIES PRODUCES AN EGG. THEY ALSO PRODUCE THE HORMONES ESTROGEN AND PROGESTERONE. THE OVARIES ARE COVERED BY A LAYER OF CELLS CALLED THE EPITHELIUM. ALTHOUGH TUMORS THAT DEVELOP IN THE EPITHELIUM TEND TO BE BENIGN, MOST OVARIAN CANCERS START IN THESE CELLS.

materials is carcinogenic. Tampons do not contain asbestos. And according to the U.S. Food and Drug Administration, the trace amounts of dioxin—which is similar to chlorine—in some products are safe and pose no health risks. We certainly wouldn't discourage women from using tampons, if that's their choice.

Some research suggests that hormone replacement with estrogen only—ERT, estrogen replacement therapy—is a risk factor for ovarian cancer. Studies have shown, for example, that women who took estrogen for more than 10 years were twice as likely to develop ovarian cancer as those who never used the hormone. The risk tripled for women who were on ERT for more than 20 years.

The link between ERT and ovarian cancer is controversial, but the research data are becoming more consistent. In the meantime, we advise our patients who are experiencing menopausal discomforts to take the smallest effective dose of any form of hormone replacement therapy for the shortest possible time to manage their symptoms. According to published data from the Women's Health Initiative, hormone replacement offers no health benefits other than relief of menopausal discomforts and prevention of osteoporosis. But it does have risks. Specifically, the combination of estrogen and progesterone raises the risk of breast cancer, coronary heart disease, stroke, and embolism.

In fact, in February 2004, the National Institutes of Health stopped the estrogen-only phase of the WHI study. By then researchers had determined that after nearly seven years of use, estrogen did not lower the risk of coronary heart disease, though it did raise the risk of stroke.

CAUSES

Some experts believe that since the risk of ovarian cancer rises in proportion to the number of times a woman ovulates, the epithelial cells may sustain genetic damage as a result of the repeated self-repair that occurs following release of an egg with each monthly cycle. If a woman starts ovulating early, never gets pregnant, and doesn't take oral contraceptives, her ovaries go through the process of injury and repair more often over the course of her lifetime. And if the growth-controlling genes in a cell undergo some type of mutation, it gets passed along through the cell division process, eventually causing cancer.

Another evolving theory focuses on the role of the hormone progesterone in protecting against ovarian cancer. Pregnancy, for example, raises the level of progesterone. Among its many actions, the hormone triggers the death of damaged cells.

Some researchers have noticed how surgical procedures that block access to the ovaries, like tubal ligation and hysterectomy, seem to lower ovarian cancer risk. This suggests the involvement of an environmental factor in triggering or advancing the disease process. As we point out to our patients, the ovaries in a sense are exposed to the outside world. The route by which sperm travel toward the egg, from the cervix through the uterus into the fallopian tubes, is the same route by which toxins could gain access to the ovaries.

Diet also may be a factor in ovarian cancer. Women who were born to immigrants from Japan, which has a low incidence of ovarian cancer, and who live in the United States develop the malignancy at the same rate as women who were born in this country. Researchers suspect that the higher risk may stem in part from the "Americanization" of the women's eating habits, which probably aren't as healthy as those of their mothers.

SCREENING

During your annual pelvic examination, your doctor carefully feels your ovaries for abnormal changes in size and contour. The ovaries are small and located deep in the pelvis, so detecting unusual growths and cysts may be difficult. Unfortunately, none of the available screening tests is accurate enough for use in the general population.

The two tests that you'll read about on the following pages, transvaginal ultrasound and CA-125, pick up benign conditions as well as cancers. Since these tests cannot diagnose cancer, a positive result requires further evaluation, and possibly surgery, to make a definitive diagnosis. In most cases, the abnormality turns out to be benign.

The high false-positive rate of these tests—particularly in pre-menopausal women—does make them impractical, not to mention anxiety-provoking, for the general population. They're expensive, too: A sonogram costs between $350 and $750; the blood test for CA-125, about $75.

Nevertheless, if you are at high risk for ovarian cancer, the possibility of a false alarm may be of less concern to you than the benefits of early detection. According to a consensus statement from the National Institutes of Health, women who have one first-degree relative—a mother, sister, or daughter—with ovarian cancer may choose to undergo screening. If you decide to have these tests, please remember: An abnormal result does not mean that you have cancer. In our practices, some of our patients opt for screening, while others decline. We think it's a very personal decision, which is why we recommend that you discuss the pros and cons with your doctor.

Women who have two or more first-degree relatives with ovarian cancer should receive genetic counseling so that they're fully informed about genetic testing. And if a woman has inherited a mutated BRCA gene, the consensus statement from the NIH recommends an annual pelvic exam, a blood test for CA-125, and transvaginal ultrasound—even though no hard evidence has confirmed that screening lowers the death rate from ovarian cancer. The Cancer Genetics Studies Consortium follows a similar guideline, suggesting that women at high risk for ovarian cancer begin screenings between ages 25 and 35 and repeat them once or twice a year.

TRANSVAGINAL SONOGRAPHY

The word *sonography* refers to the use of high-energy sound waves to create an image of an internal organ—in this case the ovaries, fallopian tubes, and uterus. The sound waves come from an instrument inserted into the vagina; hence the word *transvaginal.* The test can detect any abnormal mass, thickening, cyst, or enlargement in the ovaries, as well as any changes in bloodflow characteristic of tumor growth.

As mentioned earlier, transvaginal sonography is not a diagnostic tool. It cannot distinguish a cancer from another type of abnormality. Still, it's a quick, painless test that is more effective than a pelvic exam for spotting any unusual growths.

TUMOR MARKERS

About 80 to 85 percent of women with epithelial ovarian cancer have elevated levels of CA-125, a protein that comes from certain cells in the blood. In fact, doctors commonly use a test that measures the amount of CA-125 circulating in the body to assess how women with ovarian cancer are responding to treatment. It's much like the PSA test that's given to men who are receiving treatment for prostate cancer.

But CA-125 falls short of being a reliable marker for ovarian cancer in healthy women who have not gone through menopause. This is because levels of the protein can rise in response to many normal situations and benign conditions. For instance, both menstruation and pregnancy can increase production of CA-125. Likewise, levels of the protein may rise in the presence of endometriosis and pelvic inflammatory disease, as well as with disorders that don't involve the reproductive tract, such as liver and kidney failure and cancers of other organs.

Ironically, levels of CA-125 may not appear high in the early stages of ovarian cancer. According to one study, more than half of women with stage I ovarian cancer had normal amounts of the protein in their blood.

For all its shortcomings, CA-125 currently is the best available marker for ovarian cancer. If a blood test revealed an elevated level of the protein in a woman at high risk for ovarian cancer, her doctor probably would do further evaluation with transvaginal sonography.

Scientists are conducting studies to determine how blood tests for CA-125 might best support early detection of ovarian cancer. For instance, several measures of the protein to show the rate at which it's rising may be more useful than a single measure. Or perhaps CA-125 will turn out to be a more accurate marker for postmenopausal women.

Other trials currently under way throughout the world will assess the benefits of using both the blood test for CA-125 and transvaginal sonography. Right now, researchers at 10 medical centers across the United States are recruiting women to participate in the Prostate, Lung, Colon, and Ovarian (PLCO) Screening Trial. Sponsored by the National Cancer Institute, this large clinical trial has set out to determine whether certain tests can reduce the death rates of four major cancers in people over age 55. For ovarian cancer, the screening tests under evaluation include a regular physical exam, a blood test for CA-125, and transvaginal ultrasound.

Scientists also are looking into whether substances in the blood besides CA-125 might function as markers for ovarian cancer. One that's of particular interest is LPA (lysophosphatidic acid), a growth factor involved in the development of ovarian epithelial cells. Then there's the recent discovery of a unique protein pattern in the blood of women with early-stage ovarian cancer. Unlike CA-125, this particular pattern allowed scientists to detect the disease in every woman who had it. But the same pattern also appeared in women with benign cysts, which led to some false-positive results.

The field of proteomics, which involves the analysis and cataloging of every protein in the body, offers enormous potential for the development of new screening and diagnostic tools for conditions like ovarian cancer. But it is a new science, and its use in detecting ovarian cancer requires much more study.

PREVENTIVE STRATEGIES

Although most women who develop ovarian cancer were not at high risk for it, much of what we know about preventing the disease comes from studies of women whose chances of getting it were greater than normal. For this reason, we recommend certain "baseline" preventive strategies for all women, and then add on for those in the high-risk category. The objective of research throughout the world is to determine whether the steps that appear to lower the chances of ovarian cancer in women at high risk can do the same for women at low risk, who make up the majority of cancer patients.

DIET

Although eating lots of "plant foods"—particularly fruits and vegetables that contain vitamins A and E and beta-carotene—is thought to reduce the chances of developing ovarian cancer, the protective effect appears to be modest. A study that evaluated data collected from the more than 80,000 participants in the Nurses' Health Study found that the nutrients made no significant difference in the incidence of ovarian cancer.

On the other hand, the data did show that women who ate at least 2½ servings of fruits and vegetables every day as teenagers experienced a 50 percent reduction in their risk for ovarian cancer, which is quite significant. This finding seems to support the theory that to get the most health benefit from fruits and vegetables, everyone should eat abundant amounts of them from an early age.

But don't let this discourage you from maximizing your produce consumption now. Fruits and vegetables supply so many important nutrients that they're essential to any disease-fighting, health-promoting diet. We advise our patients to aim for at least five servings of fruits and vegetables every day—and the more, the better.

Dietary fat may influence ovarian cancer risk as well, although more study is necessary to determine how great the impact might be. For one study, published in 2002, Italian researchers compared the diets of more than 1,000 women with ovarian cancer and nearly 2,500 who were cancer-free. The women with high intakes of healthy fats from olive oil and oils made with sunflower seeds, maize (corn), peanuts, and soybeans were less likely to have ovarian cancer than those who didn't use much of these oils in their cooking. Mixed-seed oils, butter, and margarine did not affect cancer risk.

While healthy fats may help protect against ovarian cancer, we believe that too much dietary fat—especially the kind that comes from animal sources—could be a risk factor for the disease. An analysis of data from eight studies that tracked the fat intakes of more than 8,000 women linked large amounts of dietary fat—including animal fat and saturated fat—to a 24 percent increase in ovarian cancer risk. Animal fat seemed especially unhealthy, with high intakes correlating to a 70 percent increase in risk.

We should point out that while this analysis established a link between dietary fat and ovarian cancer, other studies have not found a correlation between a reduced fat intake and a decline in cancer risk. So dietary fat as a risk factor remains unproven.

Calcium is generating a lot of interest for its potential to help protect against several kinds of cancer. A 2002 study involving more than 1,000 women found that calcium from dairy sources, especially low-fat milk, could reduce ovarian cancer risk. The women in the study who consumed at least one serving of dairy a day were 57 percent less likely to develop ovarian cancer than those who drank milk less than once a week. Neither supplements nor plant sources of the mineral, such as kale, produced the same protective effect.

ORAL CONTRACEPTIVES

Studies have shown that women who took oral contraceptives containing both estrogen and progestin for at least 3 years reduced their ovarian cancer risk by about 50 to 60 percent. What's more, their risk remained low for a number of years after they stopped taking the Pill.

According to some estimates, the protective effect of oral contraceptives kicks in after 4 to 6 years of therapy. One study of women with strong family histories of ovarian cancer found that after 5 years of taking the Pill, they were as likely to develop cancer as women at low risk for the disease.

While we don't know exactly how oral contraceptives help prevent ovarian cancer, recent animal studies have shed some light on the phenomenon. It appears that progestin—a synthetic form of the hormone progesterone—causes the death of cells in the outer covering of the ovaries. This would include any abnormal cells that might become malignant. More research is necessary to answer some critical questions: Are low-dose pills as effective as high-dose pills in preventing ovarian cancer? At what age should a woman begin taking oral contraceptives? And how long must she continue treatment to achieve the desired protective effect?

If you are at high risk for ovarian cancer, talk with your gynecologist about whether oral contraceptives might be helpful for you. Keep in mind that if you inherited a mutated BRCA gene, taking the Pill may increase your risk for breast cancer. If you plan to have children, you can take oral contraceptives until you try to become pregnant, and then go back on the Pill after childbirth.

PREVENTIVE SURGERY

According to one report, as many as 1,000 cases of ovarian cancer each year could be prevented if all women over age 40—even those at low risk for ovarian cancer—who must undergo a hysterectomy were to have an oophorectomy at the same time. (*Hysterectomy* refers to the surgical removal of the uterus, while *oophorectomy* is the surgical removal of the ovaries.) Today only about half of the women in this situation have both procedures.

We always advise our hysterectomy patients who are over age 45 to consider oophorectomy as well. It could reduce their risk of ovarian cancer by at least 90 percent, if not more.

For women who do not need a hysterectomy for any medical reason, a prophylactic, or preventive, oophorectomy is an extreme solution. But it may be a reasonable choice for someone who is at high risk for ovarian cancer, particularly if she has completed her family and she's fearful and anxious about the disease.

In the mid-1990s, the National Institutes of Health called a meeting of experts to discuss prophylactic oophorectomy. The consensus of those in attendance was that the surgery should be recommended for women at high risk who had completed their families or who were age 35 or older. But given that at the time the risk reduction was thought to be about 50 percent, the Cancer Genetics Studies Consortium—organized by the National Human Genome Research Institute—did not feel comfortable making a similar recommendation based on the available research. Since then, studies have shown that the risk reduction after oophorectomy may be higher. In one study, risk dropped by 85 percent.

It is important to understand that removal of the ovaries and fallopian tubes does not guarantee protection against ovarian cancer. In cases where cancer appeared after prophylactic oophorectomy, the theory is that the disease had spread to surrounding tissue before the ovaries were removed, but it wasn't detectable at the time.

If you are considering this procedure because you carry a mutated BRCA gene, you may want to ask your doctor whether you're a candidate for hysterectomy as well. The reason is that with removal of your uterus, you would eliminate the risk of uterine cancer that accompanies tamoxifen, a chemopreventive drug for breast cancer that you may choose to take in the future.

In general, we advise our younger patients who've inherited the mutated BRCA1 or BRCA2 gene to either take oral contraceptives or consider tubal ligation, in which the fallopian tubes are closed to keep an egg from reaching the uterus. Studies have shown that either method of preventing pregnancy reduces ovarian cancer risk. Once these women pass 40, we recommend oophorectomy with or without hysterectomy.

CHEMOPREVENTION

We've seen great research interest in the potential for nonsteroidal anti-inflammatory drugs (NSAIDs) to protect against ovarian cancer. As explained in chapter 6, these drugs inhibit the COX-2 enzyme, allowing for the death of abnormal cells. With regard to ovarian cancer, they may have another preventive action as well, in that some—such as indomethacin and acetaminophen—appear to inhibit ovulation.

Chemoprevention researchers tracking large groups of women say that their findings are provocative enough to warrant further investigation. In one study, for instance, women who took aspirin at least once a week for 6 months were 25 percent less likely to develop ovarian cancer than those who took aspirin rarely, if at all. Another study found that women who took acetaminophen every day were 61 percent less likely to develop ovarian cancer than those who didn't.

Another exciting area of chemoprevention research involves the use of retinoids such as fenretinide (4-HPR). In studies to evaluate whether fenretinide could prevent a recurrence of breast cancer, the researchers discovered by chance that the drug significantly lowered the incidence of ovarian cancer.

Two collaborative research ventures—the Gynecologic Oncology Group and the Specialized Programs of Research Excellence (SPORE) in Ovarian Cancer, both sponsored by the National Cancer Institute—are conducting several clinical trials to evaluate the effectiveness of chemo-preventive drugs for ovarian cancer. Among the drugs under investigation are oral contraceptives, COX-2 inhibitors, and retinoids, such as fenretinide. In the SPORE trials, treatment with chemopreventive drugs will be followed by prophylactic oophorectomy. This will allow microscopic examination of the ovaries to determine whether the drugs produced any particular changes in the epithelial cells. Other studies are exploring the use of combinations of chemopreventive drugs, such as oral contraceptives and fenretinide.

Many of these clinical trials include measures of various biomarkers, substances circulating in the bloodstream that indicate the presence of cancer. By monitoring these markers, investigators can assess the effectiveness of a particular treatment.

WHAT YOU CAN DO NOW TO PREVENT OVARIAN CANCER

1. Eat at least five, and preferably nine, servings of fruits and vegetables every day.

2. Eat at least three servings of low-fat or nonfat dairy foods every day.

3. Limit your total fat intake by cutting back on animal and saturated fats. Use olive oil and seed oils instead.

4. Maintain a healthy weight, even if that means restricting calories to do so.

5. Be sure to get a pelvic examination every year. If you are at high risk for ovarian cancer, your doctor may recommend exams every 6 months.

6. If you are under age 40 and at high risk for ovarian cancer, talk with your doctor about taking oral contraceptives.

7. If you are over age 45 and you need a hysterectomy for any reason, ask your doctor whether you'd be a candidate for oophorectomy as well.

8. If you have a family history of ovarian or breast cancer, consult a genetic counselor to explore the possibility of genetic testing.

9. If you've inherited a mutated BRCA1 and/or BRCA2 gene, talk with your doctor about having transvaginal ultrasound and a blood test for CA-125 once or twice a year, starting between ages 25 and 35.

10. If you know that you're carrying a mutated BRCA1 and/or BRCA2 gene, and if you've completed your family or you're age 35 or older, ask your doctor about preventive surgery such as tubal ligation or oophorectomy with or without hysterectomy.

CHAPTER 13

PANCREATIC

CANCER

• • • • • • • •

As cancers go, pancreatic cancer is one of the deadliest, with an average survival time of only 3½ months after diagnosis. Although it accounts for only 2 percent of cancer diagnoses each year, it's responsible for 5 percent of all cancer deaths. That's because pancreatic cancer produces few if any noticeable symptoms in its early stages. What's more, it quickly progresses, readily invades surrounding organs like the liver, and is very resistant to available treatments.

Considering the lethal characteristics of pancreatic cancer, many experts believe that prevention—particularly by giving up smoking, which is a contributing factor in 3 of every 10 cases—offers the best hope for controlling the disease. Generally, though, preventive measures are in need of further study.

During the last century—specifically from 1920 to 1978—the incidence of pancreatic cancer tripled. Since then the number of people diagnosed in the United States each year has slowly declined, while in Europe the incidence has continued to rise.

Estimates for 2004 suggest that over the course of the year, as many as 31,860 people will learn they have pancreatic cancer. About 31,270 people will die of the disease.

Men develop pancreatic cancer more often than women, though the incidence in women was climbing for several years. Recently, that trend has slowed. As of 2004, pancreatic cancer was the 10th most common cancer among men, and the 9th most common in women. The incidence and death rate are about 50 percent higher among African-Americans than among Whites.

Between 75 and 95 percent of pancreatic cancers begin in the ducts. The rest of the chapter focuses primarily on this, the most common type, called pancreatic ductal adenocarcinoma. Among the other, very rare types of pancreatic cancer is islet cell cancer, which occurs in the cells that produce insulin.

ARE YOU AT RISK?

1. ARE YOU OVER AGE 60? Eighty percent of people with pancreatic cancer are between 60 and 80 years old.

2. DO YOU SMOKE? Smoking more than doubles the risk of pancreatic cancer and is responsible for about one-third of deaths from the disease. The risk rises with the number of cigarettes a person smokes.

3. DO YOU HAVE A FAMILY HISTORY OF PANCREATIC CANCER? Having a parent or sibling with the disease triples your risk. A family history of colorectal or ovarian cancer increases risk, too.

4. DO YOU HAVE, OR DOES ANYONE IN YOUR FAMILY HAVE, AN INHERITED SYNDROME? The word *syndrome* refers to a cluster of cancers or other conditions that result from an inherited genetic mutation. Hereditary nonpolyposis colon cancer, breast or ovarian cancer associated with a mutated BRCA2 gene, atypical multiple mole-melanoma syndrome, ataxia-telangiectasia syndrome, Peutz-Jeghers syndrome, and hereditary pancreatitis are syndromes with a connection to an increased incidence of pancreatic cancer.

5. ARE YOU OVERWEIGHT AND SEDENTARY? Studies have shown that obesity and a sedentary lifestyle may account for 15 percent of pancreatic cancer cases. People who are overweight are 72 percent more likely to develop the disease than those of normal weight.

6. DO YOU HAVE A POOR DIET? A diet that contains an abundance of fruits and vegetables, fiber, folate, and vitamin C appears to help protect against pancreatic cancer. On the other hand, cancer risk rises for those who overindulge in calories; dietary cholesterol; carbohydrates, including refined sugar; nitrosamines, found in bacon and other cured meats; and fried foods. We should mention that so far research has not proven that dietary fat raises cancer risk. Nor, apparently, does drinking coffee or alcohol.

The Pancreas

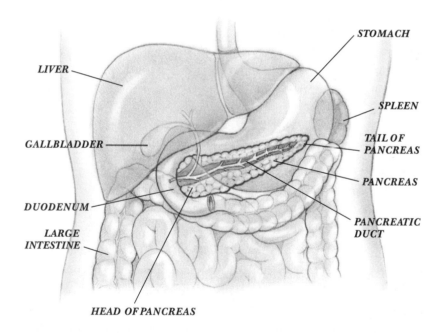

FIVE TO 6 INCHES LONG, THE PANCREAS LIES DEEP WITHIN THE ABDOMEN, JUST BEHIND THE STOMACH AND OTHER ABDOMINAL ORGANS. IT HAS TWO IMPORTANT FUNCTIONS: IT SECRETES SEVERAL HORMONES—AMONG THEM INSULIN, WHICH REGULATES SUGAR METABOLISM—AND IT RELEASES ENZYMES THAT HELP DIGEST FATS AND PROTEINS.

7. DO YOU HAVE EITHER TYPE 1 OR TYPE 2 DIA-BETES? Although pancreatic cancer is more common in people with diabetes, this chronic medical condition is not necessarily a risk factor. The chances of getting pancreatic cancer appear to be greatest in the first few years after diabetes is diagnosed, leading some experts to speculate that in some people diabetes may be an early symptom of pancreatic cancer rather than a cause.

8. DO YOU HAVE CHRONIC PANCREATITIS? People with this condition, which involves inflammation of the pancreas, have a 4 percent chance of developing pancreatic cancer over a 25-year period. By comparison, the lifetime risk is 40 percent for people with the inherited form of pancreatitis.

CAUSES

Several genetic mutations are thought to contribute to pancreatic cancer. By examining pancreatic tumors, researchers have determined that mutations occur in three types of genes: tumor suppressor genes, oncogenes, and repair genes.

The nature and impact of the mutations vary from one type of gene to the next. For instance, when tumor suppressor genes sustain damage, they may not be able to perform their job, which is to keep cells from growing out of control. Research suggests that damage to one particular tumor suppressor gene, p16, plays a role in 80 percent of pancreatic cancers.

Similarly, a mutation can activate oncogenes, allowing the transformation of normal cells into malignant ones. In about 95 percent of pancreatic cancers, an oncogene called K-ras has been altered. As for repair genes, a mutation may prevent them from correcting damage to the DNA in cells. An estimated 4 percent of pancreatic cancers involve mutations in the repair genes.

The big unanswered question is, what initiates these diverse genetic changes? Smoking may be to blame for about a third of them, while fewer than 10 percent result from inherited factors. Inflammation, like the kind in chronic pancreatitis, could be a major contributor to the cancer process. Whether specific foods or nutrients play a role remains unknown.

SCREENING

Currently, no screening tests for pancreatic cancer are available. Research has identified a biomarker called CA19-9 in the blood of people with the disease. Periodically measuring this marker can help monitor patients' progress or response to treatment. But testing for CA19-9 in healthy people still is considered experimental because it could generate too many false-positive results.

PREVENTIVE STRATEGIES

Many people who develop pancreatic cancer have none of the risk factors mentioned above. Still, if you do have any of the avoidable risk factors, you should take steps to minimize their impact.

Most important, if you smoke, quit. Research has proven that smoking raises pancreatic cancer risk. Once the carcinogens from cigarette smoke enter the bloodstream, they travel to other organs, including the pancreas. There they cause damage to the DNA in cells.

Smoking more than two packs of cigarettes a day for more than 20 years is known to cause serious gene mutations in pancreatic cells. A study published in 1999 in the journal *Cancer* looked at pancreatic cells from people who were heavy smokers and those who were moderate smokers or nonsmokers. None of the study participants had cancer at the time. The researchers identified genetic mutations associated with cancer in nearly 40 percent of the cells from the heavy smokers. Cells from the other group showed none of those mutations.

This study offers a good example of how genetic changes may precede an actual malignancy. It also shows how the more you smoke, the more likely it is that your cells will suffer genetic damage.

While we cannot cite specific studies linking physical activity to reduced cancer risk, the relationship between a sedentary lifestyle and pancreatic cancer suggests that regular exercise may have some sort of protective effect. For a variety of health reasons, not just cancer prevention, we agree with the American Cancer Society's recommendation to engage in at least 30 minutes of moderate physical activity 5 or more days per week. Aiming for at least 45 minutes of moderate-to-vigorous activity 5 or more days per week is even better.

According to preliminary research, aspirin therapy may help prevent pancreatic cancer. In 2002, researchers at the University of Minnesota published an analysis of data from an ongoing health study of 40,000 women between ages 55 and 69. The analysis showed that over the course of about 7 years, the women who took aspirin six or more times a week were 60 percent less likely to develop pancreatic cancer than those who never took aspirin. Taking aspirin once a week or less resulted in a risk reduction of about 25 percent. Nonsteroidal antiinflammatory drugs, such as ibuprofen, did not have the same impact on cancer risk.

Of course, more research is necessary to prove aspirin's protective effect. But this study certainly raises interest in using aspirin therapy as a preventive measure. For now, we don't recommend a daily dose of aspirin to lower the risk of pancreatic cancer because of the preliminary nature of the study results and the potential side effects of aspirin.

CHEMOPREVENTION

At the moment, no human studies of chemopreventives for pancreatic cancer are under way. Several substances have shown promise in test tube and animal studies; no doubt these will be the focus of future research involving people at high risk for the disease. Possible chemopreventives include the COX inhibitors, which are proving effective in preventing other types of cancer as well. (To learn more about how COX inhibitors interfere with the cancer process, see chapter 6.)

What You Can Do Now to Prevent Pancreatic Cancer

1. If you don't smoke, don't start. If you do smoke, quit.

2. Maintain a healthy body weight. (If you're not sure what's healthy for you, refer to the height/weight chart on page 225 as a guide.)

3. Eat at least five, and preferably nine, servings of fruits and vegetables every day.

4. Take a brisk walk or engage in some other physical activity most days, and ideally every day, of the week.

CHAPTER 14

CERVICAL

CANCER

• • • • • • • •

AFTER YEARS OF HOLDING THE TOP SPOT as a cause
of cancer deaths among women in the United States, cervical cancer
has fallen to 13th place, reflecting a decline in death rate of more than
70 percent. The number of cervical cancer diagnoses also dropped
more than 70 percent between 1950 and 1970. And between 1970 and
1995, both the incidence and the mortality rate fell by more than 40
percent.

These statistics demonstrate that we're making headway in the fight
against cervical cancer, thanks in large part to the widespread use of the
Pap smear, which can identify preinvasive lesions as well as invasive cancers. In fact, early detection of preinvasive lesions is far more likely these
days, particularly in women under age 50. And when it's caught early, cervical cancer is among the most treatable of all cancers.

Despite all this good news, estimates for 2004 suggest that as many as
10,520 women will test positive for cervical cancer, and about 3,900 will
die from the disease. Although screening is on the rise, the incidence of
cervical cancer remains higher for African-American women (18.6 per
100,000) than for White women (13.6 per 100,000)—possibly because
African-Americans still have less access to medical care.

In most areas of the United States, cervical cancer is twice as common among Hispanics as non-Hispanics, with an especially high incidence in first-generation migrants. What's more, the death rate from the disease is about 40 percent higher for Hispanics. One reason is inadequate screening among the Hispanic population. Another is that like African-Americans, Hispanics tend to have less access to medical care than Whites. Cultural perspectives on screening play a role, too.

ARE YOU AT RISK?

1. HAVE YOU EVER HAD A HUMAN PAPILLOMAVIRUS (HPV) INFECTION? Most sexually active women develop an acute HPV infection sometime in their lives. For the majority, the infection goes away and never leads to cervical cancer. On the other hand, virtually every case of cervical cancer results from HPV infection.

Of the more than 100 types of HPV, 30 are sexually transmitted. Some of these are known as high-risk types because they can lead to chronic infection and thus are more likely to cause cervical cancer than others. The high-risk types include HPV-16, HPV-18, HPV-33, HPV-35, and HPV-45. Of these, HPV-16—which affects about 20 percent of adult women—is responsible for most precancerous and malignant cervical lesions.

2. DID YOU BECOME SEXUALLY ACTIVE AT OR BEFORE AGE 16? The younger a woman is when she becomes sexually active, and the more sex partners she has, the more likely she is to become infected with HPV. This raises her cervical cancer risk.

3. DO YOU PRACTICE SAFE SEX? Women who have unprotected sex, especially with multiple partners, are at increased risk for HPV exposure.

4. HAVE YOU HAD ANOTHER SEXUALLY TRANSMITTED INFECTION, SUCH AS CHLAMYDIA? By themselves, these infections don't cause cervical cancer. But they may interact with HPV to increase the risk of chronic infection.

5. ARE YOU HIV-POSITIVE? If so, your immune system is not functioning optimally, and your resistance to HPV infection is lower than average. Women who have HIV are more than twice as likely to develop cervical cancer as women who don't have HIV. What's more, the cancer tends to be in a more advanced stage when it's discovered.

The Cervix

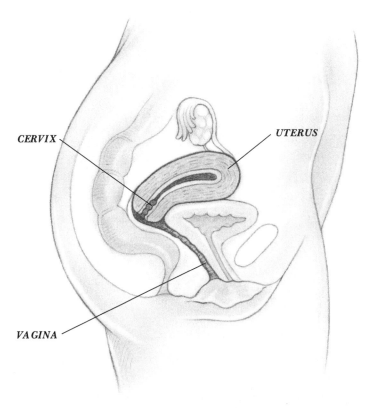

THE CERVIX IS THE LOWER, INCH-LONG NECK OF THE UTERUS, OR WOMB. IT JOINS THE UTERUS TO THE VAGINA, THEN EXTENDS INTO THE VAGINA. SPERM ENTER THE UTERUS BY PASSING THROUGH A VERY SMALL OPENING IN THE CENTER OF THE CERVIX. WHEN CANCER OCCURS, IT USUALLY BEGINS IN THE CELLS LINING THE CERVIX, WHERE THE UPPER PART JOINS THE LOWER PART. THIS IS KNOWN AS THE TRANSFORMATION ZONE.

6. DO YOU SMOKE? Women who light up are twice as likely to develop cervical cancer as those who don't. The risk appears to increase the longer a woman smokes, and the more cigarettes she smokes.

7. DO YOU HAVE A POOR DIET, WITH FEW FRUITS AND VEGETABLES? Low-income women, especially, may not eat as well as they should. Without adequate nourishment, their bodies can't fight HPV infection, which leaves them more vulnerable to cervical cancer.

8. DO YOU HAVE ACCESS TO QUALITY MEDICAL CARE? Low-income women who do not have access to good medical care, including Pap tests for early detection and treatment of precancerous cervical lesions, are at increased risk for cervical cancer.

9. DO YOU HAVE A FAMILY HISTORY OF CERVICAL CANCER? Studies point to possible familial susceptibility to HPV infection.

10. DO YOU GET REGULAR PAP TESTS? Women—including those over age 65—who do not receive regular Pap tests are between 3 and 10 times more likely to develop cervical cancer.

11. HAVE YOU BEEN TAKING ORAL CONTRACEPTIVES FOR A LONG TIME? Studies suggest that the hormonal environment in women taking the Pill is conducive to HPV infection.

CAUSES

As mentioned earlier, while most women who become infected with HPV never develop cervical cancer, almost 100 percent of cervical cancer cases are thought to result from the virus. (In men, HPV may be a risk factor for penile cancer.) Researchers believe that the high-risk types of HPV produce proteins that block the action of the cancer-fighting substances produced by tumor suppressor genes. These substances normally keep cells from reproducing too rapidly and forming cancer.

Some studies suggest that while HPV almost always is present in cervical cancer, the virus may not work alone. So-called cofactors, which are risk factors themselves, may contribute to cancer risk. Some examples:

HERPES SIMPLEX TYPE 2. Women with both herpes simplex virus type 2 (HSV-2) and HPV are two to three times more likely to develop invasive cervical cancer than those with HPV alone. No one knows why HSV-2 increases risk. According to one theory, the virus may cause inflammation that damages the DNA in cells lining the cervix. Another theory suggests that the ulcers characteristic of a herpes outbreak may allow HPV to penetrate into the tissue, where cancer develops.

CHLAMYDIA. This common sexually transmitted disease may suppress immunity and increase susceptibility to HPV infection.

HIV. HIV is a cofactor because it compromises immune function, so HPV can flourish.

SMOKING. By-products of tobacco enter the bloodstream and travel to other parts of the body—including the cervix, where they've been found in the lubricating mucus. In addition, smoking may deplete levels of vitamin C, folate, and beta-carotene, all of which seem to have a protective effect.

POOR DIET. Being undernourished may contribute to cervical cancer, possibly because the immune systems of women who don't meet their bodies' basic nutritional requirements are not be able to combat HPV infection.

SCREENING

The story of screening for cervical cancer is one of amazing success. In country after country, including the United States, the incidence of cervical cancer and the number of deaths from the disease have plummeted when screening became widely available.

In the United States, 90 percent of women age 18 or older have gotten at least one Pap test, and 60 percent have gotten a test within the past 3 years. Still, some women—particularly those without health insurance or access to medical care—are not screened as often as they should be.

To detect lesions that could lead to cervical cancer, try not to stretch the interval between Pap tests. While this kind of cancer does develop slowly, a Pap test could miss a precancer. With regular screenings, a missed lesion still can be caught before it turns into an invasive cancer.

In 2002, the American Cancer Society revised its guidelines for cervical cancer screenings to describe not only when women should begin regular Pap tests but when they could stop or alter the frequency of testing. To summarize the updated ACS guidelines:

- A woman's first cervical cancer screening should occur approximately 3 years after she initiates vaginal intercourse, or no later than age 21. (This differs from the American College of Obstetricians and Gynecologists recommendation to begin screening no later than age 18. The issue with getting a Pap test at such a young age is that it could lead to overtreatment of conditions that probably would disappear on their own. If they didn't, they still would be caught before they progressed to anything serious, provided a woman followed the ACS guideline and got her first screening no later than age 21.)

- Regular Pap tests should be repeated every year; liquid-based Pap tests, every 2 years.

- At or after age 30, women who've gotten normal results on three Pap tests in a row may reduce their screenings to every 2 to 3 years. Those with risk factors such as HIV infection or a weakened immune system may require more frequent screenings. The U.S. Public Health System Guidelines recommend a Pap test twice in the first year after diagnosis of HIV infection, then annually if the test results are normal.

- Women age 70 or older who've gotten normal results on three Pap tests in a row, and no abnormal results in the past 10 years, may choose to discontinue screening.

- Screening after a total hysterectomy—removal of the uterus and cervix—is not necessary unless the surgery was to treat a gynecologic cancer or precancer. In cases where hysterectomy involved removal of only the uterus, not the cervix, women should continue screening until age 70. The exception is when a woman's Pap tests within the previous 10 years were abnormal; then ongoing screenings are ideal.

Keep in mind that these are only general guidelines. Each woman's health history and lifestyle are different, which is why you and your gynecologist should decide how often you need a Pap test. Regular visits with your gynecologist are important. They're your opportunity to get recommended screenings—Pap tests as well as breast and rectal exams—and to discuss health matters such as contraception and self-care for cancer prevention.

PAP TEST

Named for Dr. George Papanicolaou, the Pap smear or test—also known as cervical cytology—was one of the first cancer screening tests. It also is one of the most effective. The Pap test identifies changes in cells that are shed from the lining of the cervix. It's a painless procedure that's performed during a pelvic exam. Using a tiny wooden or plastic spatula, or perhaps a specially designed brush, the physician quickly and gently wipes cells from several areas of the cervix. Traditionally, the cells were placed on a slide and examined microscopically. Today most health care providers use a liquid-based Pap test—also known as a thin-layer slide preparation—in which the cell sample is immersed in a liquid fixative.

For technical reasons, which include a more even distribution of the cells on the slide, the liquid-based Pap test is better able to detect an abnormality than the conventional test. Also, with the liquid-based test, a cell sample can be screened for HPV with what's known as reflex HPV testing.

To ensure that your Pap test is as accurate as possible, avoid getting the test during your period. And for 48 hours before the test, you should not engage in vaginal intercourse, douche, or use tampons, birth control foams or jellies, or any kind of vaginal cream or medication.

If a Pap test detects a slight abnormality, your doctor may order a follow-up test within about 4 months to confirm the results. Sometimes immediate retesting can produce a false-negative result. If a Pap test finds a more serious abnormality, or if reflex HPV testing identifies a high-risk type of HPV, your doctor will recommend a colposcopy. (We'll say more about colposcopy in just a bit.) If the HPV test turns out negative, you won't need a Pap test for another 12 months.

In one large study involving 5,000 women with mildly abnormal Pap tests, about two-thirds had abnormal cells categorized as ASCUS (for atypical squamous cells of unknown significance). The remaining third had a slightly more advanced condition known as LSIL (for low-grade squamous intraepithelial lesion). In the ASCUS group, reflex HPV testing identified almost all of the 5 to 10 percent of women with a precancer or cancer that required further treatment.

For all of its usefulness, a Pap test isn't foolproof. One of its limitations is that it has a high false-negative rate, meaning that it may fail to detect an abnormality even though abnormal cells are present. This is one reason that regular screening is so important. Precancers develop slowly, so if abnormal cells go unnoticed in one test, they may show up in the next test and still not have progressed to cancer.

HPV DNA TESTING

HPV DNA testing involves the analysis of cells from the cervix for genetic material, or DNA, from the human papillomavirus. As we explained earlier, the type of HPV determines the follow-up and/or treatment.

In May 2003, the Food and Drug Administration approved HPV DNA testing for primary cervical cancer screening. Doctors now use it in combination with the Pap test for women ages 30 and over. One reason for the age criterion is that the rate of HPV infection is very high among women under 30. If someone over 30 has HPV, it more likely is a persistent high-risk type.

COLPOSCOPY

In the event of an abnormal Pap test, a physician may take a closer look at the cervix, using a magnifying instrument called a colposcope. The procedure is known as a colposcopy. If any area appears abnormal under magnification, the physician will perform a biopsy to retrieve a tissue sample for microscopic examination.

There are several methods of performing biopsies. Your doctor will explain which of these she recommends in your case. If the biopsy detects a precancerous condition, your physician will prescribe appropriate treatment. For mild lesions, the biopsy may be all that is necessary, as your own immune system is likely to eradicate the problem. For more advanced lesions, your doctor may suggest LEEP (loop electrosurgical excision procedure), laser treatment, or a cone biopsy, which removes a larger area of tissue from the cervix than the previous biopsy. In the event that the initial biopsy finds cancer, the next step is referral to a gynecologic oncologist—that is, a gynecologist who specializes in cancer.

Of course, the ideal outcome of an abnormal Pap test is a negative result on the initial biopsy. In that case, your doctor may recommend a follow-up visit within several months for a repeat Pap test, with or without colposcopy.

PREVENTIVE STRATEGIES

Regular screenings to detect abnormal lesions and the timely removal of precancers are the most important steps in preventing invasive cervical cancer.

To reduce your risk of developing precancers in the first place, your best bet is to practice safe sex, since the human papillomaviruses that lead to abnormal cell growth and contribute to cervical cancer are spread by sexual contact. Be aware, though, that condom use alone does not completely protect against HPV infection. This is because the virus can be anywhere in the male genital area.

Although the types of HPV that cause visible genital warts do not lead to cancer, we still recommend removing the warts. Those outside the vagina, such as on the labia or around the rectum, can be effectively treated with drugs like podophyllotoxins (Condylox) and imiquimod (Aldara). Those inside the vagina require different treatment—perhaps cryotherapy, cautery, or laser therapy.

Of course, if you smoke, quit. Smoking increases cervical cancer risk in women with HPV infection. Even if you test negative for HPV, lighting up carries too high a price tag for your reproductive function and overall health. Besides, quitting smoking will reduce your chances of other types of cancer, not to mention heart disease.

In large studies, fruits and vegetables—being rich sources of vitamins A, C, and E and carotenoids—appear to offer some protective effect against cervical cancer. One member of the carotenoid family, beta-carotene, may be especially helpful because it breaks down to form retinoic acid, which regulates the growth of the type of cell that lines the cervix. This doesn't mean that you should get your beta-carotene in supplement form. Choose the whole food, the carrot or the squash, over the pill or capsule.

Research has shown that women who eat lots of vegetables high in certain nutrients—including vitamin A, beta-carotene and other carotenoids, and a form of the antioxidant lycopene—are 50 percent less likely to have persistent HPV infections. This translates to a lower cervical cancer risk.

Eating a well-balanced diet that includes fruits and vegetables also is essential to maintaining a healthy immune system. This may help prevent HPV infection.

CHEMOPREVENTION

Several trials have investigated the chemopreventive potential of nutrients such as beta-carotene, vitamin A derivatives called retinoids, folic acid, ascorbic acid, and the phytoestrogen indole-3-carbinol, or I3C. (Phytoestrogens are natural forms of estrogen from foods.) The most promising of these trials involve I3C, which comes from cruciferous vegetables like cabbage. In three small studies, abnormal cervical cells in women who took supplements of I3C showed significant improvement. In some of the women, the abnormalities disappeared completely.

More studies to evaluate the protective effects of I3C currently are under way. In the meantime, we suggest increasing your consumption of cruciferous vegetables rather than taking supplements. For now, the long-term safety of these supplements—especially in large doses—remains unproven.

The biggest news from the front line of cervical cancer prevention is a vaccine to protect against HPV-16, the virus that's responsible for half of all cervical cancers. Until recently, vaccines have been primarily for treating cancers such as melanoma. But this one actually is a preventive.

In November 2002, researchers from the University of Washington in Seattle published the results of a study that used the HPV vaccine in a large group of women. The new vaccine consists of genetically engineered particles that, while not causing an infection, so closely resemble the real virus that they prompt a person's immune system to mount a defensive attack. Once primed by the look-alike particles to search and destroy HPV, the immune system can respond to the real virus quickly and efficiently.

Of the more than 1,500 young women who completed the 17-month study, none of the 768 who received three shots of the vaccine tested positive for HPV-16 infection. By comparison, 41 of the 765 who had been given a placebo vaccine did become infected, with nine showing precancerous changes as a result of the infection. Twenty-two of the women who had received the real vaccine did develop cervical lesions that could lead to cancer, but the lesions were not associated with HPV-16.

According to an editorial in the *New England Journal of Medicine*, which published the study, "The vaccine not only prevents the disease from developing, but also prevents the (virus) from residing in the genital tract where it can infect new sexual partners." The author concludes by saying that we could see the end of cervical cancer in our lifetime.

What still isn't known is how long the antibodies produced by the vaccine will last, and whether vaccines to act against other types of HPV linked to cervical cancer will be as effective. In the study, the vaccine did not appear to have a protective effect if HPV-16 infection already was present when the woman got her shots.

Vaccines are in development that hopefully will prevent infection with other types of HPV. But many questions about these vaccines remain unanswered. For instance, should only girls get them? Or only boys? Or maybe both?

WHAT YOU CAN DO NOW
TO PREVENT CERVICAL CANCER

1. Follow the American Cancer Society guidelines for cervical cancer screening with a Pap test.

2. Practice safe sex by using a diaphragm, condom, and spermicide.

3. Eat at least five, and preferably nine, servings of fruits and vegetables every day. Be sure to include foods rich in vitamins A, C, and E, beta-carotene, and lycopene, as well as crucifers like cabbage, which are rich in the potentially protective phytoestrogen I3C.

4. If you smoke, quit.

CHAPTER 15

ORAL

CANCERS

• • • • • • • • •

CANCER CAN OCCUR IN ANY TISSUES of the mouth and throat. But when experts refer to "oral cancer," usually they mean a malignancy of the lips, gums, or tongue; the lining of the cheeks; the floor of the mouth under the tongue; or the hard or soft palate. Sometimes the oropharynx—the area of the throat just behind the mouth, including the back of the tongue and the tonsils—develops cancerous lesions. Most lesions, though, appear on the tongue, the floor of the mouth, or the soft palate.

Nearly all oral cancers are squamous cell carcinomas. Squamous cells are the ones that line the mucous membranes and structures inside the mouth.

Like most cancers, oral cancer is most common in people over age 40. But a growing number of young people are getting it, particularly on the tongue. In the 1970s and early 1980s, the incidence of oral cancer in those under age 40 rose by 64 percent. Although it has been stable since then, it remains high. There is no single, certain explanation for the increase, though the chewing of tobacco and the smoking of marijuana may be factors.

The gap between the sexes is narrowing as well, perhaps because tobacco and alcohol use among women has been on the rise over the decades. As of 2004, oral cancer ranked as the ninth most common cancer in men, affecting about 3 percent of the male population. The disease is twice as common among African-Americans as Caucasians.

Overall, the number of people newly diagnosed with oral cancer each year began to decline in the 1990s. For 2004, experts project that 28,260 Americans will develop oral cancer or cancer of the pharynx, and 7,230 would die from these malignancies. Unfortunately, the 5- and 10-year survival rate remains low—about 50 percent for all stages of oral cancer. One reason is that early detection hasn't gotten any better in at least 25 years. Oral cancers and precancerous lesions continue to go unnoticed in their earliest stages, when they're most treatable.

ARE YOU AT RISK?

1. ARE YOU A MAN? Men are twice as likely as women to develop oral cancer, though as mentioned above, the gender gap is closing.

2. ARE YOU OVER AGE 45? About 90 percent of oral cancers occur in people over 45. The incidence may be highest in older adults because the disease develops slowly, over several decades, as a number of contributing factors interact with one another.

3. DO YOU SMOKE? Smoking cigarettes, cigars, and pipes—as well as chewing tobacco and dipping snuff—accounts for 80 to 90 percent of oral cancers. The disease is four to five times more common in smokers than in nonsmokers, and cancer of the lip is especially common in pipe smokers.

4. DO YOU USE SMOKELESS OR SPIT TOBACCO? Although oral cancer risk is lower than for smokers, it still is high. A study of women who used snuff pegged their risk at four times higher than normal.

5. DO YOU CONSUME MORE THAN 30 ALCOHOLIC BEVERAGES A WEEK? Moderate to heavy drinkers are three to nine times more likely to develop oral cancer than people who consume little or no alcohol. Those who drink heavily also tend to eat poorly, and nutritional deficiencies can contribute to oral cancer.

6. DO YOU SMOKE *AND* DRINK? The combination appears to be especially hazardous, in terms of oral cancer risk.

7. HAVE YOU HAD ORAL CANCER BEFORE? People who survived their first bout with oral cancer have 20 times the average risk of developing a second oral cancer within 5 to 10 years. Despite this fact, a 2002 study funded by the Department of Veterans Affairs found that over one-quarter of people with head and neck cancers continued to smoke, most of them puffing through more than a half pack a day!

8. HAVE YOU EVER HAD A HUMAN PAPILLOMAVIRUS (HPV) INFECTION? Both HPV-16 and HPV-18—the same types of sexually transmitted virus that have been implicated in cervical cancer—

The Oral Cavity

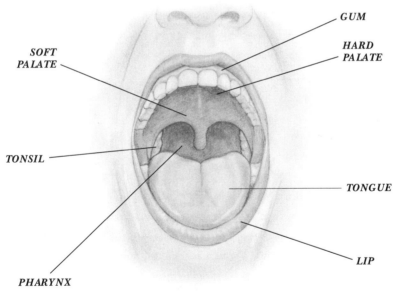

SOFT PALATE

GUM

HARD PALATE

TONSIL

TONGUE

PHARYNX

LIP

ORAL CANCER CAN AFFECT ANY STRUCTURE OF THE MOUTH. IT IS ESPECIALLY COMMON ON THE TONGUE, THE FLOOR OF THE MOUTH, AND THE SOFT PALATE. THE EARLY SIGNS OF CANCER ARE SUBTLE; SOMETIMES THEY RESEMBLE ANOTHER COMMON PROBLEM, SUCH AS A COLD SORE. IF CANCER CELLS REACH THE LYMPH NODES IN THE NECK, THEY CAN SPREAD TO OTHER PARTS OF THE BODY.

also can occur in the throat, raising the risk of oral cancer. Tests have found HPV-16 in as many as 22 percent of oral cancers, and HPV-18 in 14 percent.

9. HAVE YOU SPENT A LOT OF TIME IN THE SUN? Prolonged or frequent sun exposure raises the risk of cancer of the lip, particularly the lower lip.

10. HAVE YOU HAD WHITE OR RED PATCHES IN YOUR MOUTH? Usually these signs of irritation—called leukoplakia and erythroplakia—are benign, but about 5 percent are precancers that can develop into malignancies within 10 years. In fact, they are one of the early signs of oral cancer for which you should be alert.

11. DO YOU HAVE GUM DISEASE? People with inflamed or infected gums are four times more likely to have oral cancer than people with healthy gums.

12. DO YOU HAVE HUMAN IMMUNODEFICIENCY VIRUS (HIV) OR ACQUIRED IMMUNODEFICIENCY SYNDROME (AIDS)? Oral cancer is one of several cancers to which people with HIV or AIDS are susceptible, possibly because these infections suppress immunity.

CAUSES

Researchers have yet to pinpoint a single cause of oral cancer. The general consensus is that several factors interact to damage the DNA in cells lining the oral cavity, causing the cells to become malignant.

Infectious organisms—bacteria and viruses—may play a role in some cases because the incidence of oral cancer is higher in those with gum infections and HPV. But by far the most common culprits are tobacco and alcohol. The combination of the two elevates risk even more than either one alone, suggesting a synergistic or exaggerated effect. For example, alcohol may help the cancer-causing substances, or carcinogens, in tobacco gain access to cells.

Among these cancer-causing substances are nitrosamines, which are 100 times higher in tobacco than in bacon (perhaps the best-known source of nitrosamines). Then there's nicotine, which is addictive as well as carcinogenic. And it isn't just cigarettes that are addictive: Chewing tobacco delivers two to three times as much nicotine as smoking a cigarette.

Some researchers suspect a common thread between lung cancer and oral cancer, both of which increase with tobacco use. For example, a protein that causes the growth of lung cancer cells in heavy smokers also is present in the cells of people with head and neck cancers. In studies, the amount of this protein—called gastrin-releasing peptide, or GRP— was five times greater in the tissues of people with cancer than in those who were cancer-free. In the future, we may be able to treat lung cancer or oral cancer—or both—by eliminating or blocking GRP.

With all the emphasis on the relationship between smoking and oral cancer, it's important to acknowledge that about 25 percent of people who develop the disease are not smokers and have no other risk factors. In these cases, poor nutrition more than likely plays a role, since studies have shown that diets low in fruits, uncooked vegetables, and fiber-containing foods such as legumes and cereals increase the risk of pharyngeal cancer.

SCREENING

Researchers at UCLA are working on a computer chip that will detect certain proteins in saliva, indicating whether a person has an oral precancer or cancer. This "laboratory in a chip" will be a major breakthrough in oral cancer screening. But until it's available, most doctors and dentists must rely on their trained eyes to find early-stage cancers. The importance of this visual exam can't be overemphasized, since 85 percent of oral cancers are visible. Unfortunately, in a survey of 240 physicians practicing in Maryland, only 24 percent performed oral cancer exams on their patients age 40 or older.

One dental expert recommends keeping a flashlight in your bathroom and inspecting your own mouth once a month for any abnormal changes in your teeth or gums. And while you're checking on them, make note of any sores that bleed easily or don't heal, and any changes that affect the tissues of your mouth. Do you see any lumps, thickenings, crusting, rough spots, red or white spots, or small ulcers? Do you feel any pain, tenderness, or numbness in your mouth or lips? Even a sore that doesn't hurt could be a precancer or cancer.

As mentioned earlier, about 90 percent of oral cancers occur on the floor of the mouth, the sides of the tongue, or the soft palate. Since inspecting these areas yourself can be a challenge, ask your dentist to look for any spots, patches, or sores inside your mouth as part of your regular dental exams. Or make sure that oral cancer screening is part of your cancer-related checkup, which you should have every year if you're over age 40, according to American Cancer Society guidelines. (The National Cancer Institute recommends more frequent screenings for those who are at high risk for oral cancer.) If the exam turns up anything suspicious, a biopsy—which involves retrieving a tiny amount of tissue, using a special brush or scalpel—can diagnose or rule out cancer.

Of course, if you develop a sore that doesn't heal, a white or red patch that doesn't go away, or a lump anywhere in your mouth or on your lips, don't wait for your annual screening. See your doctor or dentist right away.

PREVENTIVE STRATEGIES

Using tobacco in any form and drinking alcohol are the two most significant risk factors for oral cancer. They also are the most avoidable. By taking control of these harmful habits, not only will you reduce your risk of oral cancer, you will also improve your chances of avoiding many other chronic medical problems.

Good oral hygiene helps protect against periodontal disease, a known risk factor for oral cancer. This means keeping teeth free from plaque—which harbors bacteria—through daily brushing and flossing and regular professional cleaning. Some researchers suspect that the bacteria in plaque may play a role in causing cancer.

A nutritious diet that includes plenty of fruits and vegetables may help lower the risk of oral cancer even in people who smoke and drink.

In 2002, a very interesting study from Greece—where smoking and alcohol are common but the incidence of oral cancer is among the lowest in Europe—found fewer cancers in people who ate more fruits, cereals, dairy products, and olive oil. These foods supply an abundance of riboflavin, iron, and magnesium, which the researchers suspected could be responsible for the protective effect of the diet. They concluded that the diet—a classic Mediterranean one—seems to prevent oral cancer.

Two years earlier, a study in the United States determined that smokers who ate more fruits and vegetables had a much lower risk of developing abnormal cells in their mouths than those who ate few of these foods. Breads, cereals, and dairy foods offered modest protection against abnormal cells as well.

In the late 1990s, researchers in Italy found that people who drank more than 20 alcoholic beverages a week but ate 13 or more servings of green vegetables a week were less likely to develop oral cancer than those who ate fewer than 7 servings of green vegetables a week. While this study shows the benefits of a healthy diet, we don't recommend such heavy alcohol consumption. The same goes for smoking: We would never endorse it, even for people who eat healthfully.

CHEMOPREVENTION

Because removing abnormal cells from the mouth with a scalpel or laser can be impractical, if not impossible, chemopreventive drugs—whether taken orally or applied topically—are an appealing alternative. Researchers have experimented with several substances, and studies continue on those that show the most potential. Currently, though, no one substance has earned wide acceptance as an effective chemopreventive for oral cancer.

For many years, the most promising method of chemoprevention involved vitamin A—including derivatives of vitamin A known as retinoids, and beta-carotene, which the body converts to vitamin A. Much of the research focused on leukoplakia because so often these white patches turn into oral cancer.

These drugs appear to be helpful in healing leukoplakia, making the spots go away or shrink. All too often, however, the patches come back. Perhaps the cells become resistant to the retinoids. Or maybe whatever is fueling the cancer process—smoking or drinking, for example—continues, so other abnormal cells develop and form precancerous lesions. Then, too, unpleasant side effects have been an issue in studies involving high oral dosages of retinoids.

One promising possibility is a form of vitamin A called acitretin (Etretin), a retinoid that doctors currently prescribe to treat psoriasis. In a small study involving 21 men and women, researchers placed acitretin tablets directly over the lesions. Seventy-one percent of those who used the drug showed marked improvement in their leukoplakia, with no side effects.

Another exciting area of research in oral cancer chemoprevention is the use of drugs that block the COX-2 enzyme, which plays a role in the cancer process. In a 2002 study, researchers from the New England Medical Center injected laboratory mice with oral cancer cells and then fed food laced with the nonsteroidal anti-inflammatory drug celecoxib (Celebrex) to some of the animals. According to the researchers, celecoxib impeded new blood vessel growth, which is necessary to feed a growing tumor. The tumors that did form were smaller than those that appeared in the mice who didn't receive celecoxib. The drug slowed cancer cell growth as well.

In 2003, Norwegian researchers determined that people with oral precancers and cancers produced more of the COX-2 enzyme than people with healthy gums. Now this research team is conducting a study to determine whether blocking the COX-2 enzyme with celecoxib prevents cancer in people with leukoplakia.

That same year, Italian researchers published an analysis of three studies, in which they concluded that people who had taken aspirin for other medical problems for 5 years cut their risk of mouth and throat cancer by two-thirds. Like celecoxib, aspirin blocks the COX-2 enzyme.

In the United States, two clinical trials currently under way at 10 medical centers are evaluating the effects of celecoxib and another NSAID on precancerous lesions in the mouth. If these trials show a benefit, much larger trials will follow to determine whether using drugs to block the COX-2 enzyme is better than the current recommended, surgical treatments for leukoplakia.

The downside of NSAIDs and other COX-2 inhibitors is that they may cause gastritis and other gastrointestinal side effects, as well as inflammation of the lining of the esophagus. These seem especially common in heavy drinkers.

Some preliminary studies suggest that natural substances such as green tea, soy, and curcumin (a compound in turmeric) may help treat precancers in the mouth. These are interesting possibilities, but more research is necessary before we can recommend drinking green tea, snacking on soybeans, and eating curry (which is seasoned with turmeric) to reduce the risk of oral cancer. On the other hand, these are healthy foods that probably won't cause any harm, if you wish to try them.

WHAT YOU CAN DO NOW TO PREVENT ORAL CANCER

1. Stop smoking. That includes cigarettes, cigars, and pipes.

2. Do not use spit tobacco products like chewing tobacco or snuff.

3. Limit alcohol consumption to no more than two drinks a day if you are a man and one a day if you are a woman. A drink equals 12 ounces of regular beer, 5 ounces of wine, or a cocktail made with 1½ ounces of 80-proof distilled spirits.

4. Protect your lips from the sun by coating them with a sun-blocking lip product.

5. Eat at least five and ideally nine servings of fruits and vegetables every day.

6. Practice good oral hygiene by brushing at least twice a day and flossing at least once.

7. See your dentist regularly for professional teeth cleanings and gum exams.

8. Get an oral cancer screening from your doctor or dentist at least once a year if you are over age 40, and every 3 years if you're younger.

9. Examine your own mouth—including your gums and tongue, the area under your tongue, the inside of your cheeks, and the hard and soft palates—once a month. If you notice any red or white patches, see your doctor or dentist right away.

PART III

YOUR
CANCER

PREVENTION PLAN

• • • • • • • • •

*I*n many ways, cancer prevention is now where heart disease prevention was more than 2 decades ago. In 1981, a landmark meeting on heart disease prevention led to the development and approval of cholesterol-lowering drugs. While the drugs are reserved for those whose lipid levels are high, the lifestyle interventions for reducing heart disease risk—get regular exercise, eat a low-fat, low-sodium diet, and maintain a healthy weight—are available to anyone. Though, truth be told, they probably are taken most seriously by those who feel they're especially vulnerable to heart trouble—perhaps because a parent suffered a heart attack or stroke, for example.

Only recently has cancer prevention received the same level of research interest and generated comparable lifestyle recommendations for risk reduction. For decades the war on cancer concentrated almost exclusively on understanding the cause and finding a cure. But then in 1964, when the link between cigarette smoking and lung cancer surfaced, the focus began to shift. Nevertheless, nearly 3 more decades passed before significant progress on the prevention front finally occurred.

In the late 1990s, research confirmed that cervical cancer results from a sexually transmitted virus—like smoking, a controllable cancer risk factor. In 1998 came reports that the drug tamoxifen could reduce the chances of breast cancer in high-risk women by as much as half. Then in 1999, the Food and Drug Administration approved celecoxib for people with familial adenomatous polyposis, a condition that greatly increases the risk of colorectal cancer. Most recently, in spring 2003, a study of nearly a million Americans determined that overweight—also a controllable risk factor—could account for as many as 14 percent of deaths from cancer among men and 20 percent of deaths among women.

PREVENTION COMES OF AGE

The time for cancer prevention certainly has arrived, as scientists continue to explore the possibilities for keeping cancer at bay or, at the very least, bringing it to an early end. While much remains to be learned, the optimal lifestyle for cancer prevention already has become apparent.

You can live your life in a way that minimizes damage to your DNA, the starting point of cancer. You can take steps to improve your personal risk profile, regardless of your genetic heritage. In the case of many specific cancers, you can get regular screening tests to detect the disease at an early and treatable stage. And as with heart disease, you may be a candidate for drugs that further reduce your cancer risk.

In the chapters ahead, we will present a cancer prevention plan that we believe will not only improve your cancer defenses but also lower your susceptibility to a host of other age-related health problems. (As you may recall from chapter 1, age is the most significant cancer risk factor.) We have synthesized the key recommendations from the previous chapters into seven basic steps that can help anyone stay cancer-free.

Changing your lifestyle to prevent cancer may be a challenge, especially if you smoke or you're overweight or sedentary. But if you can muster the motivation to stay the course with your health makeover, you will see concrete benefits. According to a 2003 report from the Institute of Medicine, the number of cancer deaths would decline by one-third over the next 12 years if people would quit smoking, maintain a healthy weight, engage in regular physical activity, and get routine screening tests. By 2015, the report concludes, the number of cancer diagnoses would drop by 100,000, and the number of cancer deaths by 60,000.

THE PROCESS OF CHANGE

So where do you begin? We suggest reading the next seven chapters, each one a step in the optimal cancer prevention lifestyle. We already have set the big-picture goals for you, and we will explain how and why they're important. Then it's your job to come up specific, doable tasks that will help achieve those goals.

As an example, let's consider the goal of maintaining an ideal weight, which many of our patients have identified as one of the greatest challenges in their lives. While you will need to gather information, such as what your ideal weight is and which program can help you get there, your most important strategy—and perhaps your first one—is to scrutinize your personal food preferences and dietary patterns. Look for unhealthy habits that you may be able to improve.

For some people, simply paying more attention to portion sizes or eating fruit instead of candy to satisfy a sweet tooth can make a remarkable difference in their ability to slim down. We also have found that counseling can help, especially for those who naturally seek comfort in food.

Of course, not everyone chooses weight control as the top priority. Ask yourself which of the seven steps in our cancer prevention plan would be hardest for you. Giving up smoking? Practicing safe sex? Making an appointment for a colonoscopy? Whichever is your top choice, it likely will require the most interim tasks to get there.

Don't be surprised if you need time to contemplate just what a particular step would demand of you before you pursue it. For example, if you spend the better part of every evening propped in front of the TV set, you have an unhealthy habit to kick, just like someone who's giving up cigarettes. Perhaps you decide to go cold turkey—canceling the cable service, selling the TV, and using the money to buy a treadmill. Or maybe you respond better to a reward system: For every 5 pounds you lose, you get to watch ½ hour of TV a day.

The idea here is to spend some time figuring out what you must do to incorporate every step of our cancer prevention plan into your lifestyle. Many of our patients have told us that tracking their progress in writing helps them stay on track. Try keeping a notebook, writing down which steps you should concentrate on and how you intend to accomplish them, as well as your successes and slipups in pursuit of an improved cancer risk profile and a generally healthier life.

Take a moment to consider how you accomplished certain goals in the past. Let's say you needed to learn a new skill for your job. It probably took time, patience, and a lot of practice. But ultimately it paid off. Can you find something in the experience that would translate to your new goal of eating more fruits and vegetables or walking for ½ hour every day? When you get right down to it, adopting a healthier lifestyle really isn't so different from other changes that may seem like second nature by now.

Do you thrive on the support and encouragement of others? Perhaps you can recruit your spouse or a neighbor as an exercise buddy. Do you have a competitive streak? Then announce to your family that by your birthday next year, you will have lost 20 pounds. You may want or need to lose even more than that, but by going slow and steady—dropping ½ to 1 pound a week—you're much more likely to keep off the pounds for the long term.

This brings us to an important point: Setting realistic goals is vital to the success of any lifestyle change. If you go on such a stringent diet that you lose more than 50 pounds in a year, that extra weight is very likely to come back. Remember, you probably didn't gain all those pounds in a single year, so you shouldn't rush losing them.

One final word of advice: Never give up. After all, change takes time. According to some experts, you need at least 3 months and sometimes 6 to make a new habit stick. During that period, you will slip up on occasion. You'll pick up a hamburger and fries at the drive-thru because you're too busy to make dinner. You'll skip the gym after work to meet friends for drinks. You'll play a great game of tennis only to realize that you forgot to put on sunscreen. Rather than berate yourself for these slips, think of them as part and parcel of the process of change, and perhaps a cue to try just a little bit harder. Eventually, your new habit will become second nature, too.

QUIT

SMOKING

• • • • • • • • •

WHETHER YOU'RE A TWO-PACK-A-DAY SMOKER or you only occasionally light up, the most important thing you can do to extend your life is stop smoking. And don't even think about just "cutting back." According to the Centers for Disease Control and Prevention, a recent large study showed that reducing tobacco use by half had no effect on the incidence of smoking-related deaths among people who continued to smoke 15 or more cigarettes a day.

Smoking cigarettes not only deposits tar, carbon monoxide, and other harmful chemical compounds—many of them known carcinogens—directly into your lungs, it also delivers a hefty dose of addictive nicotine into your bloodstream. By one estimate, the average smoker gets about 109,000 doses of nicotine a year. So in addition to damaging your lungs by inhaling irritating, carcinogen-laced smoke, you're continually depositing a known cancer promoter into your body.

While this chapter targets people who smoke cigarettes, our recommendations also apply to those who smoke cigars and/or pipes as well as to those who use smokeless tobacco, such as snuff. Smoking cigars, for example, can cause lung cancer just as smoking cigarettes does. In addition, cigar smokers are 4 to 10 times more likely to die from oral, laryngeal, or esophageal cancer than nonsmokers. While most cigar smokers don't inhale, those who do are 39 times more likely to die from laryngeal cancer than nonsmokers.

Incidentally, even nonsmokers are at increased risk for cancer just by spending time in close proximity to those who light up. This is because they're breathing in smoke that has been exhaled (called mainstream smoke), as well as smoke that comes from the end of the cigarette, cigar, or pipe (sidestream smoke). In the process, they expose their lungs to more than 60 carcinogenic chemical compounds. In 1986, the U.S. Surgeon General announced that involuntary, or passive, smoking—that is, breathing in secondhand smoke—could cause lung cancer in healthy nonsmokers.

BREAKING FREE FROM NICOTINE

Nicotine is believed to encourage cancer growth by preventing the natural death of damaged cells. When researchers exposed lung cells grown in the laboratory to nicotine, the natural process by which defective cells self-destruct stopped within minutes. This means that damaged cells not only survive, they continue to divide, and develop potentially harmful genetic changes that contribute to cancer.

Since nicotine is an addictive substance, quitting smoking can be as difficult as giving up heroin or cocaine. Many people try several times before they succeed. In fact, two-thirds of smokers are not successful in their first attempt to stop. And women appear to struggle more than men.

If you've tried unsuccessfully to quit, don't beat up on yourself or tell yourself that you'll never be smoke-free. You need to recognize that you are dealing with a physical and psychological dependency.

Within hours of your last cigarette, you probably will feel irritable and restless. You may develop a headache. And for several days or weeks, you may be hungrier, lack mental focus, and not sleep well even though you seem to be more tired than when you were smoking. Recent research shows that for smokers who quit, even the perception of time changes. Specifically, time seems to slow down, which is one reason that you may become impatient during the first few days.

Because nicotine is a mood-controlling substance, you may feel depressed, angry, anxious, or frustrated—or all of these emotions at once—when you quit. Then, too, you must contend with the many behaviors that you may associate with smoking. These ordinary behaviors act like triggers, compelling you to reach for a cigarette. For instance, some people find themselves wanting to smoke whenever they pick up a ringing telephone. Others are accustomed to lighting up after dinner or when settling down to work at the computer. These situations present unique challenges with which soon-to-be ex-smokers must learn to cope.

4 Ways to Stay Smoke-Free

Much research has focused on determining what might help smokers kick the habit. By evaluating these studies, we've learned some things that may help you in your efforts to quit.

You probably have known a few smokers who suddenly decided that they didn't want to be chained to their cigarettes any longer. So they tossed the last pack from their pockets or purses, and that was the end of it. But this scenario is rare, so don't pressure yourself to follow suit. Your chances of success are much better if you plan ahead for the difficulties of breaking a nicotine addiction.

Once you make the decision to quit, the U.S. Surgeon General suggests following four basic steps to maximize your chances of success. Here's our advice for using them to your advantage.

GET READY. Choose the date that you will quit. Then get to work on clearing your home, your car, and your pockets and/or purses of cigarettes and matches. Give away all of your ashtrays, too. They'll only encourage other people to smoke around you, which you don't want.

GET SUPPORT AND ENCOURAGEMENT. Telling your family, friends, and coworkers about your quit date is helpful. But lining up additional support online, by telephone, or through a smoking cessation program really increases your chances for success.

Several national organizations offer information and advice to people who want to quit. Among the best resources:

- American Cancer Society—(800) ACS-2345 or www.cancer.org
- National Cancer Institute—(877) 44U-QUIT or http://cis.nci.nih.gov/fact/3_14.htm
- American Lung Association—www.lungusa.org

Your local hospital, church, or health club may sponsor a smoking cessation program. Nicotine Anonymous is another option. Once you start looking, you'll find support groups are everywhere.

LEARN NEW SKILLS AND BEHAVIORS. Overcoming a smoking dependency is a two-part process. There's ending your physical and psychological addiction to nicotine, and there's reining in the ritual of lighting up, putting the cigarette in your mouth, and inhaling deeply. So quitting for good involves not only coping with nicotine withdrawal but also learning new habits to replace the old, reach-for-a-cigarette ones.

Initially, you may want to find things to occupy your body and mind so you're too busy to smoke. Exercise of any kind—perhaps walking, cycling, swimming, or lifting weights—is a good choice because it serves a dual purpose. First, it relieves tension and distracts you from the urge to light up. And second, it helps control your weight.

It isn't unusual for smokers to gain up to 10 pounds after they quit. For some reason, the extra weight is more likely to show up in women than in men. While it may be common, it isn't "normal." You need to be careful not to trade one health risk (smoking) for another (obesity).

Since you probably will want to nibble on snack foods as an alternative to putting a cigarette in your mouth, plan ahead by stocking up on a variety of bite-size fresh fruits and vegetables. Keeping a glass or bottle of water with you at all times also is helpful. It occupies your hands and mouth, and as a bonus, it doesn't supply any calories.

Another good idea is to practice some form of stress reduction—deep-breathing exercises, for example. Some ex-smokers have said that the only time they took a really deep breath was when inhaling from a cigarette. So practice exhaling, pushing as much air from your lungs as you can. Then on your next inhalation, completely fill your lungs with fresh oxygen.

Meditation—in which you sit quietly for 15 or 20 minutes and concentrate on your breathing, on counting, or on a particular word—helps calm frayed nerves and relieve tension. Taking a hot bath at the end of the day can be equally relaxing, as can doing slow stretches or practicing yoga.

To help break free from a cigarette habit, the American Cancer Society offers the four A's:

- *Avoid* being around people who tempt you to smoke or in situations where smoking occurs.

- *Alter* your daily habits. For example, take a walk after lunch instead of grabbing a cup of coffee, which could prompt you to light up.

- Find *alternatives* to putting a cigarette in your mouth, such as chewing sugarless gum, sipping on bottled water, and eating raw vegetables or sunflower seeds.

- Engage in *activities* that occupy you and help distract you from smoking.

GET MEDICATION AND USE IT CORRECTLY. Nicotine replacement therapy (NRT)—which is available as gum, lozenges, inhalers, nasal spray, and patches—may double your chances of quitting for good. We should note that NRT is not recommended for women who are pregnant or nursing, for women who are trying to become pregnant, or for anyone who's under age 18, smokes fewer than 10 cigarettes a day, or has a preexisting medical condition.

NRT delivers a low dose of nicotine into your bloodstream—less than you'd get from a cigarette, but enough to ease withdrawal symptoms. By reducing the dose slowly, you wean yourself from nicotine over a period of weeks or months, making not smoking somewhat easier. And while using NRT, you can work on the behavioral changes that are necessary to end the ritual of lighting up and inhaling.

According to a review of medical studies that evaluated the success rate of various NRT options, the odds of quitting successfully were best for smokers who used the nasal spray. Inhalers and lozenges were equally effective, followed by patches and then gum. For highly dependent smokers, the gum containing a 4-milligram dose of nicotine produced better results than the 2-milligram dose.

You may find that a particular form of NRT has certain advantages that appeal to you. For instance, a nasal spray provides immediate relief from withdrawal symptoms. The gum serves as an oral substitute for cigarettes, and allows you to control the dosage. The patch, on the other hand, delivers a steady, measured dose.

Some people find that using multiple forms of NRT works best for them. For example, you could wear a patch to maintain a consistent level of nicotine, and then chew the gum as needed. In studies of this combination, people have used up to four pieces of gum a day, in addition to the patch.

NRT can cause side effects, including dizziness, racing heartbeat, and nausea. These result from the nicotine; in fact, they are similar to what many smokers likely felt when they first introduced nicotine into their systems by smoking a cigarette. Relief from these side effects may be as simple as switching to another form or brand of NRT or lowering the dose.

Among the specific forms, the patch may cause redness and other signs of skin irritation. Users of nicotine gum sometimes report throat irritation, hiccups, and jaw discomfort. Taking care not to chew the gum too fast may prevent these side effects.

Like NRT, the antidepressant drug bupropion (Zyban) helps diminish nicotine cravings. It can more or less double your chances of giving up smoking for good. If NRT has not worked for you, ask your doctor about using bupropion instead. Be aware that the drug isn't appropriate for people who have seizure conditions or eating disorders, or for those who are on other medications that contain bupropion hydrochloride.

Some people find that they need both bupropion and NRT to control their nicotine cravings. Research shows that using both may be more effective than using either one alone. For this reason, we recommend using both bupropion and NRT, as well as participating in some type of behavioral or supportive therapy, to give yourself the best chance for success.

RESTORING YOUR BODY TO GOOD HEALTH

Minutes after you smoke your last cigarette, your body will begin repairing the damage of smoke inhalation and nicotine addiction. According to the National Cancer Institute, your circulation improves almost immediately, and your pulse rate and blood pressure gradually drop to normal. Within days, your sense of taste and smell return.

To maintain these benefits and improve your health, you must become a long-term former smoker. Once you've been smoke-free for about 2 years, your risk of heart attack will decline. After 5 years, your risk of cancer of the lungs, mouth, throat, and esophagus will decrease by half. After 10 years, the death rate among former smokers is similar to that of nonsmokers.

Yes, quitting smoking probably is one of the hardest things you ever will do. But 45 million people manage to do it every year, most of them on their own. If you tried to quit but couldn't, a support group or smoking cessation program may provide the structure and incentive you need. And be patient with yourself. After all, 70 percent of smokers who quit start again within 3 months. They—and you—can succeed. Proof is in the fact that since 1965, the percentage of smokers in the United States has dropped by almost half, from 42 to 23 percent.

MAINTAIN

A HEALTHY

WEIGHT

• • • • • • • • •

"As the obesity epidemic spread,
the prevalence of overweight among U.S.
adults increased by more than 60 percent."
—CENTERS FOR DISEASE CONTROL AND PREVENTION,
OBESITY TRENDS AMONG U.S. ADULTS BETWEEN 1985 AND 2001

THERE PROBABLY ARE AS MANY THEORIES to explain why we are becoming an overweight nation as there are fad diets that claim to take off those extra pounds. Even though we spend millions on diet books, products, and programs, the needle on our collective scale keeps creeping upward. And we adults aren't the only ones getting heavier. So are our children. In 1999, 14 percent of adolescents were overweight—three times the percentage of 20 years ago. And overweight adolescents have a 70 percent chance of becoming overweight adults.

If you're carrying more pounds than you should, we hope that you will consider making one very important anticancer resolution: to achieve and maintain an ideal weight. Making this commitment is essential to reducing your risk of many types of cancer, as well as most chronic diseases. And if you have children, keep an eye on their eating and exercise habits, too, so they might never need to "unlearn" unhealthy pound-producing behaviors.

FINDING WHAT'S HEALTHY FOR YOU

When we say "an ideal weight," we are not referring to the societal ideal that's perpetuated by the images of supermodels and celebrities in magazines and movies. We mean ideal from a health point of view. In general, men don't seem to equate "ideal" with "underweight," as women do. In fact, they may perceive "ideal" as a little heavier than is healthy. So whether you're a man or a woman, you may need a reality check on just what your ideal weight is. It may not be as simple as looking at a height/weight chart.

Over the past 50 years, the parameters of healthy weight have evolved. We now know that we need to consider not just how much a person weighs but also how much fat makes up that weight and where the body stores that fat.

Your doctor can use several different tools to gauge what's healthy for you. One is the traditional height/weight chart, which, despite its shortcomings, is standard in most doctors' offices. Another is body mass index (BMI), a measurement that equals your weight in kilograms (1 kilogram = 2.2 pounds) divided by your height in meters squared (39.37 inches = 1 meter). You can spare yourself the trouble of doing the math by using a computerized calculator like those available at www.consumer.gov/weightloss/bmi.htm, http://nhlbisupport.com/bmi, and www.healthfullife.umdnj. edu. Or, if you simply want to determine whether you are in a healthy range, overweight, or obese, refer to the chart on the opposite page.

Keep in mind that even if your weight falls within a healthy range, having a high percentage of body fat increases your risk of many chronic diseases, including some types of cancer. The location of body fat is important, too. As research now shows, people who store excess amounts of fat in their abdomens are at greater risk for heart disease and diabetes, and possibly cancer.

By the same token, you may fall in the overweight range according

Are You at a Healthy Weight?

To use the following chart, simply locate your height to the left of the grid and your weight along the bottom. The point at which the two intersect is your body mass index (BMI). As a general guideline, a BMI of 18.5 to 24 falls in the "healthy" range, while 25 to 29 is "overweight." A BMI of 30 or higher is an indicator of obesity.

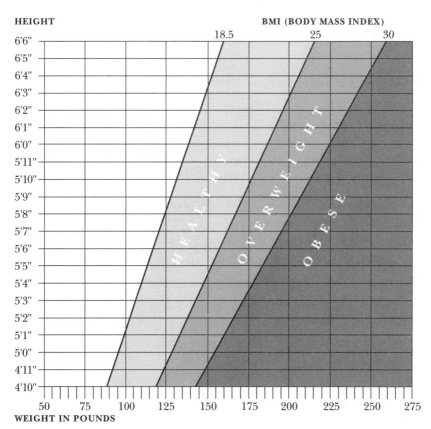

Source: Report of the Dietary Guidelines Advisory Committee on the Dietary Guidelines for Americans, 2000, page 3.

to the charts but actually be quite healthy. This is because muscle weighs more than fat, and looking at only height and weight or BMI doesn't account for body composition.

Some people like to use changes in measures of body fat to gauge the effectiveness of their exercise programs. The more muscle they build with strength training, and the more fat they lose by burning calories with aerobic exercise, the less body fat they'll store.

Certainly if you're concerned about whether you have too much body fat, you should get checked. It's a simple procedure performed by physicians, personal trainers, and nutritionists, who use a device similar to calipers to measure a pinch of skin at specific places on the body. For most people, it produces fairly accurate results.

If you are very obese or you want a more precise calculation of body fat, you need to go to a weight-loss clinic or seek out a physician who has the necessary special equipment. Some health clubs offer portable "bio-electrical impedance" devices, which are nearly as accurate as underwater weighing—considered the gold standard for body fat measurement.

WEIGHING YOUR OPTIONS

Comparing how much you *should* weigh and how much you *do* weigh is an important first step toward achieving and maintaining an ideal weight. So what's next? You need to decide what you will do to take off and keep off any extra pounds or, if you're already at your ideal weight, what you will do to stay there. Here's what we recommend.

IF YOU DON'T HAVE A WEIGHT PROBLEM
Kudos to you for keeping your weight within a healthy range! But be careful not to become overconfident. You still need to pay attention to the number of calories you consume from food, and the number you burn through exercise. Otherwise, you easily could fall victim to "weight creep," a phenomenon that becomes more common with age.

As you get older, your metabolism naturally slows. You also begin to lose muscle mass, which normally helps burn calories. This is why, as men and women move from their twenties into their forties, they gain between 1.8 and 2 pounds a year. You may find that you need to work a little harder to maintain your weight over time. Keep an eye on your waistline and the scale.

Other factors besides age—like pregnancy and parenthood, fluctuating hormones, out-of-control stress, and busy schedules that curtail physical activity and increase reliance on fast food—can contribute to weight gain as well. As a general rule, people cannot maintain an ideal weight for the long run without cutting back on calories and increasing physical activity.

If you are like most Americans, you may be getting too many of your calories from fats, oils, sugars, and refined carbohydrates. Take a step toward cancer prevention right now by clearing your cupboards of these foods and replacing them with nutrient-rich fruits and vegetables. (We'll say more about the "five a day" recommendation for fruits and vegetables, and the corresponding health benefits, in the next chapter.)

If you aren't already engaging in some type of physical activity most days of the week, we suggest turning to page 247. There you will learn how you can use exercise to increase the number of calories you burn. And the more calories you burn, the more you can take in from healthy foods without gaining weight. In this way, you can avoid extreme calorie restriction as you grow older.

Even if you currently are in the healthy range of the height/weight or BMI chart, you need to make a lifelong commitment to stay there. The best way to do it is through a combination of portion control (which we'll discuss later in the chapter) and physical activity.

We suggest monitoring your weight by stepping on the scale once a week. If you notice an extra pound or two, think about what might have caused this gain. The idea is to intervene in any behaviors that may be expanding your waistline before they become entrenched in your lifestyle.

IF YOU ARE OVERWEIGHT

Whether you've put on weight slowly, gradually moving up in pant sizes over the years, or relatively quickly, perhaps after quitting smoking, the surest route to weight-loss success is to slim down slowly but steadily. Some people prefer to jump-start their efforts with a severe calorie-restrictive diet, which can take off the first 10 or so pounds rather fast. But sustaining this type of diet can be very difficult, and often the pounds come back. It's not only frustrating but potentially unhealthy, according to some weight-loss experts.

This is why we recommend the slow-but-steady approach, beginning with portion control. Depending how much you intend to lose, achieving your ideal weight may take a year or longer. But if you take your time, you're much less likely to go up and down the height/weight or BMI chart like a yo-yo.

At the start of your weight-loss program, the one number that's more important than all the rest is how many calories you require to maintain your weight right where it is. Then you can move on to how many calories you need in order to lose those extra pounds at a healthy rate, and what sorts of foods can help accomplish that goal *and* provide important nutrients. One simple formula for determining your maximum calorie intake is to multiply your current weight by 13 if you are sedentary, 15 if you are moderately active, or 18 if you work out for at least an hour every day. Another, more precise formula involves calculating your resting, or basal, metabolic rate (BMR):

1. Multiply your current weight by 10 for your BMR.

2. Multiply this figure by 30 percent (0.30) if you're sedentary or 40 percent (0.40) if you're active.

3. Add the two numbers for your maximum calorie intake.

Let's suppose that you weigh 150 pounds and are sedentary. The math would look like this:

1. $150 \times 10 = 1{,}500$ calories (your BMR)

2. $1{,}500 \times 0.30 = 450$

3. $1{,}500 + 450 = 1{,}950$ calories per day to maintain your current weight

Eating fewer calories and getting more physical activity on a daily basis will, of course, lead to weight loss. Although you likely won't take off too many pounds through exercise alone, your level of activity does help determine the number of calories you can consume without gaining weight. For instance, a brisk 10-minute walk burns 50 calories; a 30-minute walk, 150 calories. So if you're sedentary, you're missing out on an easy way to burn the caloric equivalent of a slice of bread or a glass of milk.

Armed with this information, you're ready to start on a plan to achieve your ideal weight and maintain it. A bit later in the chapter, we'll outline some strategies that can increase your chances of success.

IF YOU ARE OBESE

Though any excess weight increases your risk of cancer somewhat, people who are extremely obese—with a BMI over 40—are most vulnerable to the disease. If you fall anywhere within the obese range, you should launch your weight-loss efforts with a visit to your doctor. She can perform a complete physical exam and help create a plan to slim down safely and sensibly. You may be facing a bigger challenge than someone who needs to lose just 5 or even 25 pounds, but being 30 or more pounds overweight is riskier for your health, too.

FEWER CALORIES = FEWER POUNDS

For the majority of people, being overweight or obese is the result of taking in more calories than they use up. Age, genetics, metabolism, and level of physical activity influence this calorie balance. But the bottom line is, if you want to lose weight, you need to eat less and exercise more.

Nevertheless, because some physical conditions—such as hypothyroidism or polycystic ovary syndrome—may contribute to weight gain, it's important to see your physician for a checkup before you try to slim down, especially if you're 30 or more pounds overweight. Certain drugs, such as some antidepressants and steroids, also can cause weight gain. So be sure to tell your doctor about any prescription or over-the-counter medications you are taking.

In general, cutting 200 to 500 calories from your daily diet and burning more calories through regular physical activity will lead to a slow but steady—and healthy—weight loss. Some popular diets advocate even lower calorie intakes, but we believe that fueling your body on 800 to 1,000 calories a day is not particularly healthy. And as mentioned earlier, sustaining extreme calorie restriction for a long period of time is nearly impossible.

We encourage our patients to count calories, at least in the beginning, and to look for simple ways to clip 200 to 500 calories from their daily intakes. It may be as simple as exchanging a bagel with cream cheese for an egg white vegetable omelet at breakfast.

This isn't a trendy diet. It doesn't ask you to give up carbohydrates or to eat only grapefruit. We're convinced that by eating real foods in sensible portions, you are more likely to take off and keep off the extra pounds. And as you learn which foods deliver the most nutrients for the fewest calories, you'll develop an eating plan that you can live with for the long term.

Calorie counting and portion control naturally go together. It seems to us that as restaurant servings have grown larger, many Americans have lost their sense of healthy portion sizes. We suggest buying a pocket-size calorie guide to carry with you at all times, as well as a small notebook to write down what you eat and how many calories the foods contain. Although keeping such close tabs on your calorie intake may seem difficult and cumbersome at first, over time you'll become familiar enough with the calorie contents of certain amounts of various foods that portion control will become second nature.

If you have access to the Internet, tracking your calories and portions is even easier and a lot more interesting. The USDA's Center for Nutrition Policy and Promotion (CNPP) has an excellent free interactive site on which you can keep a daily record of the foods you eat. Just go to www.usda.gov/cnpp and click on "Interactive Healthy Eating Index." There you can get an instant analysis of your calorie intake for the day, as well as a nutritional breakdown—from fats to vitamins and minerals—of the foods you've eaten, a healthy eating index score, and a graphic illustration of how your food choices and eating habits compare with the USDA's Food Guide Pyramid. You also can find out whether you've consumed an adequate number of fruits and vegetables, too much meat, or not enough dairy, whole grains, or fiber. It's kind of like a daily nutritional report card.

We've found that after a few weeks of conscious eating—reading labels for serving sizes and carefully monitoring portions—people develop a kind of sixth sense about their diets. They don't need to measure every morsel of food to know that they're getting just the right amount. Eating healthfully becomes second nature, and slimming down follows.

In the next chapter, you'll learn how eating lots of fruits and vegetables can protect against cancer and help lose weight, too. Of course, some people gain weight even when following a largely vegetarian diet—which shows the importance of calorie counting and portion control, even when you're making smart food choices. That said, if you've been filling up on fats, oils, sweets, and other calorie-dense foods, you may find that simply cutting back on these foods and following steps 3 and 4 of our cancer prevention plan will help get rid of any extra pounds.

ON TRACK FOR SUCCESS

While we can make general recommendations about diet and exercise, the fact is that weight loss and maintenance is a highly individualized endeavor. What works for your best friend may do nothing for you, and vice versa. The one constant for everyone is that slimming down requires a commitment to a new way of living.

Whether you work closely with your physician, enroll in a hospital-based course, or join a commercial plan like Weight Watchers, your chances of success are much greater if you participate in a structured program that teaches behavior-changing strategies such as how to read labels and how to manage stress. Such programs also provide a support network for sharing ideas and addressing challenges, which many people find helpful.

In our opinion, anything that can help achieve and maintain your ideal weight is worth exploring—not just to look better in the mirror, though that's a nice perk, but to lower your odds of cancer. A 2003 study of 900,000 men and women, published in the *New England Journal of Medicine*, highlights the impact of obesity on cancer risk. When the study began, all of the participants were cancer-free. Sixteen years later, those with high BMIs were more likely to have died from cancer.

According to the researchers who conducted the study, excess weight is responsible for 14 percent of cancer deaths in men and 20 percent of cancer deaths in women. Furthermore, they concluded that as many as 90,000 cancer deaths a year could be prevented if people would maintain a healthy weight. Clearly, to prevent obesity-related cancer deaths, the most important step you can take is to avoid being overweight in the first place.

EAT

AT LEAST

5 FRUITS

AND VEGETABLES

A DAY

· · · · · · · · ·

FOR MORE THAN A DECADE, the National Cancer Institute has been reminding us Americans to aim for "five a day"—fruits and vegetables, that is. We have made some progress toward that goal, in that we're eating at least 22 percent more fruits and vegetables today than in 1970. Still, the vast majority of us are coming up short. According to the NCI, only 23 percent of adults eat five a day, the bare minimum. Only 4 percent get nine a day, which is ideal.

The "five a day" guideline isn't just about quantity. It is also about variety. We're coming up short in that regard, too. Consider that potatoes account for half of all the vegetables that we Americans eat—and worse, they're fried half the time. Just behind them in popularity is iceberg lettuce, another nutritionally inferior veggie. Don't get us wrong; we have no problem with either food. Our concern is that they don't deliver the vitamins, minerals, and cancer-fighting phytochemicals that come from choosing a mix of colorful vegetables.

Take a moment to think about what you ate yesterday. Did you manage to get a total of five fruits and vegetables? Remember, five is the bare minimum—not the ideal, especially for cancer prevention. The truth is, we probably need nearly twice that number to reduce our cancer risk.

The National Cancer Institute recommends nine fruits and vegetables a day as optimal. The American Institute for Cancer Research says that if every American consumed 15 to 30 ounces of fruits and vegetables every day, we could reduce the incidence of cancer by at least 20 percent. And Walter Willet, M.D., Dr.P.H., professor of nutrition at the Harvard School of Public Health, recommends three to five servings of vegetables *and* two to four servings of fruits a day, based on his study of the diets of more than 100,000 Americans.

WHY YOU NEED FRUITS AND VEGETABLES

We've seen the shocked expressions on our patients' faces when we tell them about the nine-a-day recommendation. And we know how much of a challenge eating that many fruits and vegetables can be because we try to do it ourselves. But the fact is, if you want to reduce your risk of cancer, then you ought to make colorful fruits and vegetables the bulk of the 2 to 3 pounds of food you consume each day. Here's why.

THEY CONTAIN A LOT OF WATER

More water translates to fewer calories, bite for bite. So simply by eating more of these foods, you likely will take in fewer calories than if you were satisfying your appetite with foods rich in fats, oils, and sugars. The average American gets about one-third of a day's calorie intake from these calorie-dense, nutritionally devoid foods. And women are especially vulnerable to their lure, eating far more of them than men, according to diet surveys.

Fruits and vegetables are the least expensive, healthiest all-natural low-calorie food that you could find. If you're struggling to maintain a healthy weight (see step 2 of our cancer prevention plan), try substituting fruits and veggies for the high-calorie foods in your diet.

THEY ARE GOOD SOURCES OF FIBER

In recent years, the connection between fiber and cancer prevention weakened when several major studies failed to find a reduced risk of the disease among people who got healthy amounts of fiber from their diets. Then, in 2003, two important studies turned the tide again.

One study in the United States found that people who ate the most fiber—about 36 grams a day—had the fewest intestinal polyps, a risk factor for colorectal cancer. The other involved about a half million people in 10 European countries, making it the largest-ever study of the relationship between nutrition and cancer. It concluded that people who ate about 35 grams of fiber a day were 40 percent less likely to develop colorectal cancer.

The fiber in fruits and vegetables also protects against cancer by helping to maintain a healthy weight. It creates a feeling of fullness with fewer calories than foods like pasta and white bread.

Fiber takes two forms: soluble and insoluble. The soluble kind absorbs water and becomes bulky, taking up space so you feel full. It also may attach to carcinogens, toxins, and bile acids and shuttle them out of the intestinal tract.

Insoluble fiber—which comes from the skins of apples, pears, peaches, and apricots as well as the seeds of strawberries and tomatoes—acts as a kind of scrub brush in the colon. This also helps protect against exposure to carcinogens and toxins.

Most Americans consume only about half of the 20 to 30 grams of fiber a day that the National Cancer Institute recommends. If you haven't been getting enough, slowly add it to your diet, taking as long as a month to build up to 20 or so grams a day. Eating too much fiber too fast can cause bloating, gas, and stomach cramps.

The Best Fiber Sources

According to National Cancer Institute guidelines, you should aim for 20 to 30 grams of fiber a day to help reduce your cancer risk. Fruits and vegetables definitely will contribute to your fiber intake, but to make sure that you're getting enough, you need whole grains and beans, too. The following foods deliver the most fiber per serving.

FOOD	AMOUNT	GRAMS
Barley	½ cup	15.9
Bran cereal	¾ cup	12–15
Sweet corn	1 ear	6.6
Brown rice	1 cup	6.5
Kidney or pinto beans	½ cup	5–6
Grape-Nuts	½ cup	5
Potato	1 medium	4.8
Blackberries	½ cup	4.5
Rolled oats	½ cup cooked	4.5
Strawberries	10	3.8
Brussels sprouts	¾ cup	3.4

As you increase your fiber intake, don't forget to drink more water as your thirst dictates. This will help prevent constipation and keep intestinal waste moving out of your body.

While fruits and vegetables are good sources of both soluble and insoluble fiber, satisfying your daily fiber needs with these foods alone would be a challenge. To reach 30 grams, for example, you would need to eat far more than five servings of fruits and veggies a day. Four servings of fruits would supply about 11 grams, while five servings of vegetables would add another 14 or so grams. So you still would be about 5 grams short.

This is where whole grains and beans come in. One-half cup of kidney beans supplies nearly 5.5 grams of fiber. A slice of whole wheat bread contains 2.11 grams, compared with a slice of white bread, which has only 0.5 gram. One-half cup of brown rice contains 3.25 grams. (For more examples, see "The Best Fiber Sources" opposite.)

As with fruits and vegetables, we Americans tend to consume far fewer whole grains than we should. The U.S. Surgeon General recommends aiming for at least three servings a day; the national average is about one-half of a serving a day. Only 13 percent of us get even one serving a day.

THEY SUPPLY AN ABUNDANCE OF CANCER-PREVENTING NUTRIENTS

The more calories that come from refined foods like pastas, white bread, and baked goods, the lower the concentrations of vitamins, minerals, and other nutrients circulating in your bloodstream. Obviously, you have only one option for reversing this trend, and it's to eat fewer fats, oils, and sugars to make room for more fruits and vegetables. Foods that contain an abundance of fats and sugars deliver calories without nutrients, which is why you might hear them described as empty-calorie foods.

Many of the nutrients in fruits and vegetables are antioxidants, which are essential for disarming the free radicals that attack DNA. But some do double duty, assisting in the repair of damaged DNA and providing the raw material to create new DNA. Some even block the actions of cancer-causing molecules.

A number of scientists believe that we humans differ in our genetic programming for metabolizing nutrients. This would explain why our individual nutritional needs vary so much. It also may be the reason that inadequacies in a particular nutrient might lead to cancer in one person but not in another.

The medical community is just beginning to learn about these genetic distinctions. Until we understand more about them, we personally aren't comfortable recommending nutritional supplements, with a few possible exceptions. On the other hand, we don't hesitate to suggest eating fruits and vegetables. They not only are safe, but also deliver key cancer-fighting nutrients in combinations that the body can use efficiently.

One recently published study shows how ineffective nutritional supplements can be and how much we don't know about the effects of altering a person's nutrient intakes with single supplements. For this study, researchers assigned healthy men who typically ate few fruits and vegetables—2.6 servings a day, on average—to two groups. Those in one group took daily supplements of vitamin C, vitamin E, and folic acid for 90 days. Those in the other group took placebos. In blood tests, the supplement takers did show higher levels of the vitamins than the placebo takers. But when the researchers measured antioxidant activity in the men's bodies, they found no difference between the two groups. Clearly, just adding supplements is not enough. You need to eat whole fruits and vegetables, too.

Studies involving large groups of people consistently show that those who ate foods rich in vitamin C, vitamin E, and folate had a lower incidence of cancer. Beta-carotene also may bestow some protective effects, though the research hasn't been quite as conclusive. Here's what we know so far about the cancer-fighting potential of this nutritional quartet.

FOLATE. This B vitamin—found primarily in deep green leafy vegetables, asparagus, beets, broccoli, and avocados—is best known for reducing the amount of homocysteine in the blood. In this way, it helps to reduce the risk of heart disease and prevent birth defects. Now research suggests that folate also may play a role in protecting against cancer, especially colorectal cancer.

Without folate, the carbon atoms that normally attach to DNA in an orderly manner instead are in disarray, which alters the behavior of the DNA. What's more, the body isn't able to repair and manufacture nucleic acids that make up the DNA, leading to cell mutations. So as cells divide, they grow uncontrollably, setting the stage for cancer.

Both human and animal studies have linked folate deficiency to various cancers, including those affecting the breast, cervix, and lung. But the greatest evidence of folate's potential protective effect comes from a study involving more than 25,000 people. The researchers found that as folate intake increased, the incidence of colon polyps decreased.

Even if you take in 400 micrograms of folate a day, the equivalent of the Daily Value, you may not be getting enough to reduce your cancer risk. Drinking alcohol actually could rob your body of the vitamin.

Folate is so important in preventing cancer that it is one of the few nutrients for which we do recommend supplementation because you really can't meet your body's needs through foods alone. The U.S. government advises women of childbearing age to aim for 400 micrograms a day, so certainly this amount is safe.

VITAMIN E. This vitamin takes several forms, collectively known as tocopherols. They are the first line of defense in the membrane that surrounds each cell and protects the cellular contents.

Many studies involving large groups of people have shown that when the intake of vitamin E increases, the incidence of cancer decreases. But as the Alpha-Tocopherol Beta-Carotene (ATBC) Cancer Prevention study—one of the largest of its kind—found, taking supplements did not affect lung cancer risk. Some experts argue that the 50-milligram dose was inadequate. And some speculate that vitamin E supplementation is useful only for those who are deficient in the nutrient.

Nevertheless, scientists continue to explore and evaluate the therapeutic value of vitamin E. For instance, studies currently under way should help determine whether alpha-tocopherol—a particular form of vitamin E—can help protect against breast or prostate cancer.

Vitamin E is oil soluble, and so is abundant in the oils and seeds of vegetables, rather than in the whole foods. Until we see more research, we don't recommend taking vitamin E supplements for cancer prevention.

VITAMIN C. Many people take vitamin C on a daily basis, thinking that it helps prevent colds—a benefit that remains unproven. But since the mid-1960s, researchers have been studying the nutrient for its cancer-fighting potential. They have established a link between vitamin C— which is abundant in many fruits and vegetables—and a lower incidence of cancers of the oral cavity, larynx, esophagus, lung, breast, pancreas, cervix, and rectum.

Besides being a powerful antioxidant, vitamin C stimulates the immune system and prevents the activation of certain cancer-causing chemicals. For example, it converts nitrites—carcinogenic substances common in smoked meats—into harmless nitrates. In this way, scientists believe, vitamin C could prevent stomach cancer in people who smoke food to preserve it.

High-Test Fruits and Vegetables

Researchers have established markers for the free radical activity of various foods, including fruits and vegetables. By getting a generous mix of the following top choices in your diet, you can maximize your body's ability to defend itself against cancer and other diseases.

TOP 10 ANTIOXIDANT-ACTIVE FRUITS	TOP 10 ANTIOXIDANT-ACTIVE VEGETABLES
1. Prunes	1. Kale
2. Raisins	2. Spinach
3. Blueberries	3. Brussels sprouts
4. Blackberries	4. Alfalfa sprouts
5. Strawberries	5. Broccoli
6. Raspberries	6. Beets
7. Plums	7. Red peppers
8. Oranges	8. Onions
9. Red grapes	9. Corn
10. Cherries	10. Eggplant

As with vitamin E, we recommend getting vitamin C from foods—especially citrus fruits, among the best sources—rather than taking supplements.

BETA-CAROTENE. Along with lutein and lycopene (see "A Polyphenol Sampler" on page 242), beta-carotene is one of seven so-called carotenoids. It is by far the most plentiful. The body converts beta-carotene—from yellow-orange fruits and vegetables such as squash, cantaloupe, sweet potatoes, yams, carrots, and nectarines, as well as from leafy greens such as kale, chard, beet and collard greens, and spinach—into vitamin A.

Many studies have shown that the more beta-carotene people eat, the less likely they are to develop cancers of the cervix, ovary, lung, esophagus, larynx, nasopharynx (the nasal passages and the back of the throat), and oral cavity. The incidence of breast, stomach, and prostate cancers declines as well, though not by as much.

While beta-carotene is a very active scavenger of free radicals, it appears to protect against cancer in a number of other ways, such as by boosting the activity of the immune system and blocking the activation of cancer-promoting genes. In fact, animal studies using beta-carotene were so convincing that they prompted researchers to launch several large human trials of beta-carotene supplementation in the 1980s and 1990s. But the results of these trials were disappointing.

In fact, in the ATBC study—which involved smokers at high risk for lung cancer—beta-carotene supplements produced a surprisingly adverse reaction. They actually increased the risk of lung cancer.

Another study—the Carotene and Retinol Efficiency Lung Cancer Chemoprevention Trial, which examined the long-term use of beta-carotene in combination with vitamin A—ended earlier than planned. The reason: Researchers noticed a 46 percent increase in deaths from lung cancer and a 26 percent increase in deaths from cardiovascular disease among those taking the supplements, compared with those taking a placebo.

It still isn't known whether beta-carotene directly affected lung cells or if it triggered some other reaction that indirectly contributed to the cancer process. Nevertheless, the results of these two trials prompted researchers to rethink the safety and usefulness of nutritional supplements for cancer prevention. Once again, we see the importance of getting the bulk of our nutrients from whole foods—and especially fruits and vegetables—rather than relying on supplements to make up for any shortfalls.

THEY ARE RICH IN PHYTOCHEMICALS

Phytochemicals are natural plant substances that help prevent cancer through a variety of actions. Some short-circuit carcinogens in the body, while others interrupt the cancer process at a very early stage. Most do a little bit of both. In fact, an active area of research involves determining precisely how these micronutrients—with unwieldy names like glucosi-

nolates, thiocyanates and isothiocyanates, and phenols—might help reduce cancer risk.

Because this research isn't all that far along, we can't draw conclusions from it just yet. We certainly would not advise taking any of the phytochemicals in supplement form. Instead, we offer this general rule of
thumb: Eat plenty of fruits and vegetables in a variety of colors every day,
and you will get a generous mix of phytochemicals in adequate amounts
to boost your cancer defenses.

A Polyphenol Sampler

Foods contain thousands of polyphenols, including some 4,000 different
flavonoids alone. Thus far, only a handful have been the subject of extensive
laboratory and animal research. Human studies are only beginning to reveal
how these powerful antioxidants might support cancer prevention. Here's
just a sampling of the polyphenols that have gone under the microscope, so
to speak, and their possible protective effects. (*Note:* Until we know more
about the safety and effectiveness of polyphenol supplements, we recommend getting these nutrients from foods alone.)

POLYPHENOL	SOURCE	CANCER-FIGHTING POTENTIAL
Anthocyanins	Strawberries, raspberries, blue-berries, cherries, red plums, red and blue grapes, red cabbage, eggplant, beets	These antioxidants may have estrogen-like activity. In test tube experiments, berry extracts impaired blood vessel growth, which is necessary for tumor growth.
Catechins	Tea	Regular tea drinkers are less likely to develop cancers of the esophagus, lung, and stomach. The antioxidant activity of catechins, as well as a compound called epigallocatechin gallate (EGCG), may be responsible for the protective effect. While it's too soon to recommend drinking more tea to lower cancer risk, we do suggest substituting tea for coffee.

Of the phytochemicals that are generating interest as cancer preventives, polyphenols are the most abundant in our diets. We get them from fruits, vegetables, and some beverages, particularly tea and red wine.

Polyphenols come in many different forms, the names of which you probably have heard or seen in health news reports recommending that you eat more berries or tomatoes, drink green tea, or replace meat with soy products. Researchers are concentrating on this particular group of phytochemicals to understand how they might help protect against cancer.

POLYPHENOL	SOURCE	CANCER-FIGHTING POTENTIAL
Glucosinolates (indoles and sulforaphane)	Broccoli, cauliflower, cabbage, kale	The chemicals produced when these polyphenols break down help detoxify carcinogens.
Isoflavones	Soybeans	The large amount of soy in traditional Asian diets often is cited as the reason for the low incidence of breast and prostate cancers in these countries. So far, though, research is inconclusive.
Lutein	Broccoli, kale, spinach, blueberries	A large study investigating a variety of carotenoids, including lutein, determined that they reduced the risk of breast cancer in premenopausal women.
Lycopene	Red fruits and vegetables such as tomatoes, watermelon, and strawberries; cooking tomatoes in stews or sauces enhances the availability of lycopene	Research associates a diet rich in tomatoes with a reduced rate of all cancers. Of 72 studies included in a 1999 analysis, 57 found that as lycopene intake increased, cancer risk decreased. Other research has shown that this polyphenol helps prevent prostate cancer and shrink existing tumors. It also lowers insulin-like growth factor-1, a cancer promoter.
Quercetin	Apples, onions	One study identified a lower incidence of lung cancer among men with higher intakes of quercetin.

Most polyphenols are antioxidants that help disarm free radicals, preventing them from damaging the DNA inside cells. But some act like estrogens and antiestrogens, hence their name *phytoestrogens*. The daidzein and genistein in soy are examples of phytoestrogens, as are the lignans in flaxseed and flaxseed oil. Phytoestrogens have generated a lot of research activity because the incidence of breast cancer is lower in countries where the traditional diet features large amounts of soy.

All of the polyphenols vary slightly in their chemical structures, which determine how well the body absorbs them and how they interfere with the cellular changes that can lead to cancer. Because they differ from one another, the best way to get a mix of them is—of course—to eat a variety of fruits and vegetables. Variety is key because of the considerable range in polyphenol content, even for one kind of vegetable. For instance, a study comparing fresh beet greens identified a 4½-fold variation in antioxidant activity and a 3½-fold variation in flavonoid content depending on where the beets were grown. When they are harvested also affects antioxidant activity.

As researchers learn more about the cancer-fighting potential of polyphenols, individual supplements of these phytochemicals almost certainly will go on the market. We strongly caution against taking isolated polyphenols. We don't know enough about them, and what we do know raises questions about whether in large doses they could contribute to cancer, rather than prevent it.

STRATEGIES TO STRIVE FOR 9

Now that you know why you need as many as nine servings of fruits and vegetables a day, your next step is to figure out how you're going to do it. One way to eat enough of these foods without consuming too many calories is to follow the principles of the Mediterranean diet. In general, this diet emphasizes complex carbohydrates—not the refined starches and sugars that deliver calories but no nutrients—as well as colorful fruits and vegetables, olive oil, fish, and a little yogurt and cheese.

What Is a Serving?

Nine servings of fruits and vegetables a day certainly seems like a lot. But once you know the size of serving, it's not quite so daunting. You may want to copy this list to post on your refrigerator or tuck into your purse or wallet so you can keep a tally toward your daily quota. One serving equals:

- ½ cup cooked or raw vegetables
- 1 cup raw leafy greens
- 1 medium piece of fruit
- ½ cup cooked or raw fruit
- ¼ cup dried fruit
- 6 ounces fruit juice

While experts long have touted the Mediterranean diet for its ability to lower the risk of heart disease and stroke, we believe that it encompasses all the right ingredients to protect against cancer as well. The only caveat is that to accommodate all those fruits and vegetables without going overboard on calories, you may need to cut back on complex carbohydrates such as whole grain pastas and breads. Work with your menus and watch your scale until you find the right combination that allows you to maintain a healthy weight.

Keep in mind that while you want variety, it isn't necessary to eat nine different fruits and vegetables every day. Your nine servings could consist of the following: an orange and hot cereal cooked with ¼ cup of dried cherries for breakfast; an apple as a mid-morning snack; 2 cups of salad at lunch, with a cup of strawberries for dessert; a tomato juice cocktail before dinner; and a cup of salad plus either a handful of asparagus or a cup of broccoli with your dinner entrée. And if you still have room for more, how about a poached pear for dessert?

As you adjust your diet to include more cancer-fighting fruits and vegetables, don't be surprised if you start to lose weight as well. After all, most of these foods supply fewer calories than fats and sugars do, yet they're more filling because of their water and fiber content. At first you should measure your portions to avoid taking in too many calories. With practice, though, estimating serving sizes will become second nature.

While eating whole fruits and vegetables is the most straightforward approach to getting your nine a day, feel free to be more creative in incorporating these foods into your diet. If you're making whole grain waffles or pancakes, for example, stir some strawberries, blueberries, or bananas into the batter. Or whip them with yogurt for delicious smoothies. Likewise, you can mix fresh or frozen vegetables with whole grain pastas or noodles, or use them as "stuffing" for omelets or toppings for pizzas.

If you aren't a big fan of vegetables, experiment with different cooking methods, such as steaming, roasting, and broiling, which will help improve the flavors. Just be careful not to overcook—especially with boiling, as vital nutrients could leach into the cooking water.

Vegetables may be more palatable if you combine them with other foods. Besides the options above, you might try adding them to soups, stews, and sauces, which can help disguise their taste.

STEP 4

GET

MOVING

• • • • • • • • •

Nearly 200 studies have examined the effects of physical activity on cancer incidence. So far scientists have gathered convincing evidence that exercise can reduce the risk of breast and colorectal cancers. It also may protect against uterine and prostate cancers, though the research in this regard is less certain but still intriguing. So while we can't say that a sedentary lifestyle actually causes cancer, studies have confirmed for us that an active lifestyle improves the odds of avoiding some cancers.

Just how exercise might protect against cancer is a topic of investigation. From what we can tell, being physically active appears to bestow immune-boosting benefits, along with exerting a potentially positive influence on the ebb and flow of hormones that affect cancer risk. Physical activity also helps maintain a healthy weight by building muscle, which increases your metabolism, so you burn more calories. Whether you need to shed pounds or you already have achieved your ideal weight and you want to stay there, regular exercise will support your efforts.

Please don't misinterpret what we're saying. In general, exercise alone isn't enough to melt away excess weight. It will help with modest weight loss of about 5 pounds. If you want to take off more than that, you'll need to cut back on calories as well.

Plan for Fitness

Making physical activity a part of your life presents a challenge that is not so different from eating to lose weight. You know that if you cut calories, you can drop 10 or 15 pounds in a few months. But if you don't have a standby maintenance plan for when you stop counting calories, one that you can stick with for the rest of your life, you're going to regain those pounds faster than you lost them.

If you aren't careful, your fitness habits can follow much the same course. We've seen some of our patients join a gym, even spend money on a personal trainer, and get in shape amazingly quickly. Then they go on vacation, or their training sessions come to an end, and their workouts become more sporadic. Soon their fitness gains disappear, and they're back to where they started. What you need is an exercise program that suits your lifestyle—both for general fitness and for weight control.

A study from a decade ago found that 75 percent of women who maintained their weight loss for at least 2 years had integrated physical activity into their lifestyles, with most of them working out for ½ hour more than 3 days a week. Only 36 percent of those who regained their weight had been working out regularly—further proof that exercise is essential to weight maintenance.

In 2003, when the National Cancer Policy Board reviewed the literature on cancer prevention, they made various recommendations to help shape a healthier lifestyle for all Americans. The authors of the resulting report, *Fulfilling the Potential of Cancer Prevention and Early Detection*, included these practical suggestions.

1. Accumulate exercise in short bouts.

2. Make your day-to-day life more active.

3. Use exercise equipment at home.

The scientific research proves that these steps work. But in our experience, how they play out can vary tremendously from one person to the next. Some people, for instance, prefer a highly structured fitness regimen in which they engage in a vigorous 30- to 45-minute workout first thing in the morning and are done for the day. Others hate strenuous exercise but are happy to go for a brisk 3- or 4-mile walk at lunchtime or after dinner. Some prefer hopping on a treadmill in the comfort of their homes. Others like to go to a gym, where they aren't distracted by family members or a ringing telephone. We encourage you to find what works best for you.

If you've been sedentary, your initial goal should be to establish an exercise program that will get you moving most days of the week. Then, to sustain your momentum, you need to broaden your view of physical activity and find ways to make it an easy and natural part of your lifestyle.

What we're really suggesting is a two-part plan. First, choose a moderately vigorous activity that you can do on most days of the week. If you manage only 3 days a week, don't despair. It's a start. Second, make the other hours of your day more physically active. You really can't overdo, unless you push yourself too hard too soon. The beauty of this two-part plan is that you always have a backup for those days when you must skip a workout or when parking a few blocks from the office and walking to work isn't an option.

We've found several ways to squeeze more activity into our lives on a daily basis. For example, we always take the stairs when we're going only a few flights up or down. Sometimes if we take the elevator, we get off two flights before our destination and walk the rest of the way.

HOW MUCH IS ENOUGH?

Research has yet to identify a specific duration or frequency of workout that can reduce the risk of cancer. That said, various organizations—including the American Cancer Society—have come up with their own recommendations.

The ACS, for instance, suggests that adults engage in moderate activity for 30 or more minutes 5 or more days each week. Moderate to vigorous activity for 45 or more minutes 5 or more days each week may be even better, according to ACS guidelines, because it could further reduce the risk of breast and colorectal cancers.

The Centers for Disease Control and Prevention sets a slightly more modest goal: Engage in moderate-intensity activity for 30 minutes on most days, if not every day, of the week. Examples of moderate activity are walking 2 miles in 30 minutes and bicycling 5 miles in 30 minutes.

Meanwhile, the National Academy of Sciences suggests an hour of moderate exercise every day if you're trying to lose weight. If you already are at a healthy weight and you have no trouble maintaining it, then 30 minutes of moderate exercise most days should be enough to provide health benefits.

One recent study found that exercise could reverse the accumulation of visceral fat deep within the abdomen, a pattern of fat distribution that contributes to so many health problems, possibly including cancer. According to the researchers behind the study, the most significant declines in the shortest time occurred in those who engaged in large amounts of vigorous exercise, such as jogging 17 miles a week. This was the first clinical trial to examine the effects of different amounts and intensities of physical activity on visceral fat.

We believe that engaging in some type of moderate exercise for 45 to 60 minutes 2 or 3 days a week, and then taking advantage of every opportunity to be more active on the other days, is realistic for most people. The balance between intense workouts and everyday movement depends on your personal preferences. Both will build strength, burn calories, improve fitness, and help prevent chronic diseases such as cancer. No matter what the mix, the long-term goal should be to get exercise every day.

START SLOW

Once you make a commitment to a more active lifestyle, you may be tempted to jump right in, working out as vigorously as you can from day 1. But if you've been relatively sedentary for the past few years, starting too fast and doing too much could cause you to hurt yourself, burn out, or collapse in exhaustion. Whatever your current level of fitness—or lack thereof—gradually increase the intensity and/or duration of your exercise sessions so you avoid mishaps and setbacks.

If you're accustomed to walking the dog for a half hour when you get home from work, add another 5 minutes every few days. Or step up your pace and then stay at that pace for a little bit longer every few days. If you're in the habit of going straight from the dinner table to the couch, just taking a stroll around the block is a good start to a regular exercise program. Personally, we've found that we fare better when we set specific goals for ourselves—such as planning to walk for a half hour after dinner, instead of being vague and saying, "Let's try to walk more often."

We recommend that you see your doctor before starting any kind of vigorous exercise program. At the very least, get your blood pressure checked. If you're a man over age 40 or a woman over age 50, ask your doctor whether you should get an exercise stress test to confirm that your heart is healthy. This is especially important if you've been relatively inactive in recent years, if you are overweight, or if you have some other health problem. An exercise stress test also presents an opportunity to establish your safe target heart rate zone, which we'll explain in just a bit.

WHAT MAKES YOU SWEAT?

When we refer to moderately vigorous or vigorous exercise, we're talking about *aerobics*, a term coined in the 1960s. An aerobic activity is one that challenges your heart and lungs, thereby improving your fitness level. The harder you work, the faster your heart beats and the more oxygen you inhale. Any repetitive movement that uses your large muscles— walking, climbing stairs, rowing on a machine, swimming—and that increases your heart rate qualifies as aerobic.

You know that you're exercising vigorously when your heart rate reaches a point within your target heart rate zone, which is a range between 50 and 75 percent of your maximum heart rate. Staying within this zone pushes your heart and lungs enough to improve their function. It is considered safe for most healthy people.

The best way to accurately establish your safe target heart rate zone is to get an exercise stress test. Short of that, you can use a mathematical formula like the one on page 252; it uses age to calculate your target heart rate zone.

We want to make clear that your target heart rate zone is only an estimate. You still need to listen to your body. For example, if you're gasping for breath, you should slow down—even if your heart rate isn't in the range that you've calculated.

Two other methods have earned a thumbs-up from exercise physiologists as good gauges of aerobic exertion. One is the so-called talk test.

Find Your Target Heart Rate

Experts use a number of formulas to determine the target heart rate zone. The following is the simplest. But keep in mind that your zone is an estimate. What is comfortable and doable for you may be as many as 10 points higher or lower.

* Calculate your maximum target heart rate by subtracting your age from 220 if you're a man or from 226 if you're a woman.

* Multiply this figure by 50 percent to determine the lower number and by 75 percent to determine the upper number of your target heart rate zone.

For purposes of an example, let's suppose that you are a 45-year-old man. Your calculations would look like this.

* $220 - 45 = 175$

* $175 \times 0.50 = 87.5$; $175 \times 0.75 = 131.25$

Your estimated target heart rate zone is 88 to 131.

To check your heart rate during a workout, place your index and middle fingers over the artery on the inside of your wrist and count the beats for 15 seconds. Multiply the number of beats by 4 to estimate your heart rate for 1 minute. If you are at the low end of your target heart rate zone after 15 or so minutes of exercise, push a little harder. If you've passed the upper number, slow down.

Keep in mind that over time, you'll need to work a little harder to get into your heart rate zone. This is because you're getting fitter as your heart beats stronger and your lungs are able to consume more oxygen.

You know you're working hard enough when you can talk, but just barely. If you're straining to talk, you should reduce the intensity of your workout.

Another method that also has the support of many fitness trainers is what's known as the perceived exertion scale. As its name suggests, you simply rate your level of exertion on a scale of 1 to 10. For example, 5 would be moderate—how you might feel if you were walking briskly. Eight would be very hard—how you might feel if you were jogging. You can use the perceived exertion scale to monitor your workouts and make sure that you're neither pushing too hard nor slacking off. If you find your level of exertion beginning to decline, you can pick up your pace so that you're working just a little outside your comfort zone.

Whether you use target heart rate, the talk test, or the perceived exertion scale, keeping track of your workouts may help fuel your commitment to getting fit. Some of our clients keep a running log on their computers. Others write in journals, taking notes about their exercise programs as well as their eating habits.

Switching between aerobic activities can help prevent boredom, which unfortunately has derailed many a well-intentioned exercise program. For example, you might sign up for an aerobic dance class—one of the best calorie burners around—for the social atmosphere, then stick with stairclimbing on days when you feel like being alone with your thoughts or listening to music. If you prefer to exercise at home, consider purchasing a cross-country ski machine or a rower to trade off with your outdoor walks. You also might look into joining a dance club. Dancing is a great workout, and fun!

A host of books, magazines, and Web sites offer suggestions for finding a physical activity that suits your personality and your lifestyle, as well as tips for sticking with it. Experiment, have fun, and do your best to stay committed to your program for a minimum of 3 months. That's about how long you need for regular, heart-pounding exercise to become a habit.

Once you get accustomed to working out, it does seem to become addictive. Initially, the rise in endorphins—the so-called feel-good brain hormones—that occurs with exercise could be reinforcing the behavior. Over time, you'll notice improvement in your muscle tone and body shape. And if you like the way you look, you'll have extra incentive to stay fit.

DESIGNING AN ACTIVE LIFE

Building more activity into your lifestyle requires that you examine every aspect of your daily routine and ask, "How could I move more when I do this?" Taking the stairs instead of the elevator at every opportunity, as we do, is the most obvious example. But once you start looking, you quickly will identify many other opportunities for being active.

Walking to the receptionist's desk to check for phone messages after a meeting instead of picking up the phone to request them adds a few more steps—and possibly even a flight of stairs—to your day. Rather than call the corner deli to deliver your lunch, pick up your sandwich or salad yourself. Stand when you usually sit—when you talk on the phone, for example. Run errands within a 10-block radius of your home or workplace on foot instead of by car. Some of our clients have said that rather than sit in our waiting rooms before their appointments, they sign in and then take a walk around the block.

We suggest that you wear a pedometer for a week. You'll be surprised at how much you can boost the total number of steps you take each day just by forgoing e-mail and walking to your colleagues' offices to pass along information, or squeezing in a few minutes on the stairclimber whenever your favorite TV show takes a commercial break. Even doing household chores like vacuuming can add steps to your day. And consider this: taking 10,000 steps equals 5 miles and burns between 2,000 and 3,500 calories. So get moving!

PRACTICE

SAFE

SEX

● ● ● ● ● ● ● ● ●

MOST PEOPLE ARE WELL AWARE OF the relationship between sexual activity and HIV (human immunodeficiency virus) transmission. But they may not realize that HIV is a risk factor for two types of cancer: Kaposi's sarcoma and non-Hodgkin's lymphoma.

Other sexually transmitted viruses and bacteria can increase cancer risk as well. Like HIV, herpes simplex virus type 8 has a strong association with Kaposi's sarcoma. Genital herpes and chlamydia contribute to the kind of cervical cancer that results from HPV (human papillomavirus). And both hepatitis B and C increase the chances of liver cancer.

The two most reliable methods for preventing sexually transmitted diseases (STDs)—including those that can lead to cancer—are completely abstaining from oral, vaginal, and anal sex; and being in a long-term, mutually monogamous relationship with an uninfected partner. If you are beginning a new relationship, both you and your partner should get tested for STDs before you have sex. But don't interpret negative results as a green light for an unprotected intimate encounter. First, it takes as long as 3 months to develop the antibodies to HIV, which is what a screening test will detect. In other words, if you or your partner have been infected only recently, you could test negative for HIV and still carry the virus. Second, detecting HPV in men is difficult.

So until a relationship is long-term and monogamous, we suggest using a condom and spermicide, along with a woman's birth control method such as a diaphragm or an oral contraceptive. Some data suggest that oral contraceptives may allow HPV to survive, so the spermicide and condom are crucial.

And always, if you aren't absolutely sure that your partner is free from STDs or that he or she is monogamous, practice safe sex, which means using a condom every time you have an intimate encounter. If you or your partner experience any symptoms of an STD, abstain from sex until you know for certain that neither of you has an active infection.

THE BEST PROTECTION AVAILABLE

Condoms are not perfect. They are not 100 percent effective in preventing STDs that travel via bodily fluids, though the kind made from latex do greatly reduce the risk of transmission. They are even less useful in preventing STDs that occur as a result of skin-to-skin contact, such as herpes simplex and HPV.

Still, short of abstinence, condoms with spermicide are the only option for protecting against STDs. So you need to know how to use them correctly, especially if you're not in a long-term, monogamous relationship.

When buying condoms, keep in mind that the best material for stopping the spread of HPV is latex. It is less likely to break than animal membrane or polyurethane. Condoms are designed for one-time use, so each intercourse—whether oral, vaginal, or anal—requires a new condom with spermicide.

A man should try several different brands and sizes to find one that fits properly—not so tight that it is uncomfortable or can break, and not so loose that it slips off his penis. While condoms generally come in three sizes, brands do vary.

Handle the condom carefully. Don't rip open the package with your teeth or unroll the condom with your fingernails. If you have a problem with breakage, consider switching to the "extra-strength" kind, which are slightly thicker and stronger.

Some condoms come already lubricated. If you're using one that isn't, or if you need additional lubrication, choose a water-based product, such as K-Y Jelly or Astroglide. Besides being more comfortable, a lubricant can prevent breakage during intercourse. Steer clear of petroleum jelly and massage oils, which break down latex.

While the Centers for Disease Control and Prevention maintains that spermicides such as nonoxynol-9 are not effective in stopping the transmission of gonorrhea, chlamydia, or HIV, these products may help protect against HPV. They also help prevent pregnancy. For these reasons, we strongly recommend using both a condom and spermicide.

Put on the condom when the penis is erect and before any genital contact occurs. Promptly after ejaculating and while the penis still is erect, hold the condom against the base of the penis and withdraw from your partner.

Incidentally, researchers have developed a female condom that's made from polyurethane. One end is closed, with a ring that is inserted into the vagina and covers the cervix; the other end is open. Like the male condom, the female condom is for one-time use only. To date, no clinical studies have evaluated its effectiveness in preventing STD transmission. But it is an alternative when, for whatever reason, a male condom isn't appropriate. While some drugstores carry the female condom, you may have better luck finding them online.

WHY TAKE A CHANCE?

As a result of public education campaigns and increased awareness of the serious health effects of STDs, about 20 percent of adults participating in a national survey reported that they had used condoms the last time they had engaged in sexual intercourse. Unfortunately, that number has not improved since 1996, and it falls far short of the 50 percent goal established by the Department of Health and Human Services as part of its National Healthy People 2000 initiative.

The fact remains that between 7 million and 12 million adults are at increased risk for acquiring or transmitting HIV primarily because of unsafe sex. The odds of acquiring or transmitting other STDs no doubt are even greater. Factor in the possibility of developing cancer as a result of infection, and you have every reason to take steps to protect yourself. Practicing safe sex may not be foolproof, but it definitely lowers your risk.

A V O I D

O V E R E X P O S U R E

T O

S U N L I G H T

• • • • • • • • •

I N   2 0 0 2 ,   T H E   N A T I O N A L   I N S T I T U T E   of Environmental
Health Sciences added ultraviolet (UV) radiation—whether from the sun
or from an artificial source such as a tanning bed—to its list of 228
cancer-associated substances. Fortunately, this is one carcinogen against
which you can easily protect yourself. Just by wearing sunscreen and practicing other simple preventive measures, you can lower your skin cancer
risk dramatically.

This raises an important point. As helpful as sunscreens are—and
we'll explain what to look for when you buy one—it's important to remember that these lotions, creams, sprays, gels, and sticks are only the
first step in a three-step sun-protecting process. Second, you need to physically minimize your sun exposure as much as you can. Ideally, you should
avoid the sun between 10 A.M. and 4 P.M. (11 A.M. and 5 P.M. daylight saving
time), when the rays are strongest. And take extra precautions when

you're on or near a body of water, high in the mountains, or near the equator—anyplace where the sun is especially intense.

Third, when you head outdoors, be sure to cover yourself and seek shade whenever possible. Some people mistakenly believe that if they're wearing a sunscreen, they can stay out in the sun for as long as they want. True, a good broad-spectrum sunscreen will help keep the skin from burning for a few hours. But it won't be 100 percent protective. Furthermore, some evidence suggests that prolonged radiation exposure—even in the absence of sunburn—is a risk factor for skin cancer.

COVER UP BEFORE HEADING OUT

We're not suggesting that you stay indoors all day or shroud yourself from head to toe when you do venture out. Just use common sense. For example, when you go to the pool or the beach, take along an umbrella for extra shade. Cover up with a tightly woven, light-colored shirt when you aren't swimming. If you are fair-skinned, wear a shirt over your bathing suit even when you are in the water. Top off with a hat that shades the tops of your ears and the back of your neck, as well as your face. And don't forget sunglasses. They not only protect your eyes, they also shield your eyelids and the surrounding skin.

If you work outdoors or are particularly sensitive to the sun, you may need to wear a long-sleeved shirt and long pants—in addition to a hat and sunglasses—at all times. An ordinary cotton T-shirt won't be completely protective, since about half of the sun's ultraviolet rays can penetrate the fabric, even more if the shirt becomes wet. These days you can buy stylish lightweight garments made from tightly woven fabrics that offer even better protection from the sun. These clothes are becoming more widely available in specialty stores, by catalog, and online at sites such as www.sunprotectiveclothing.com, www.sunemporium.com, and www.solumbra.com.

Do you have red hair? If so, your skin has little melanin, the natural pigment that normally would help minimize sun damage. In your case,

How Sensitive Are You?

Your sensitivity to the sun varies according to the amount of natural pigment, or melanin, in your skin. The U.S. Food and Drug Administration and the American Academy of Dermatology categorize skin type in this way.

SKIN TYPE	SUN HISTORY	EXAMPLE
I	Always burns easily, never tans, extremely sun sensitive	Red-haired, freckles, Irish/Scotch/Welsh
II	Always burns easily, tans minimally, very sun sensitive	Fair-skinned, fair-haired, blue-eyed, Caucasian
III	Sometimes burns, tans gradually to light brown, sun sensitive	Average skin
IV	Burns minimally, always tans to moderate brown, minimally sun sensitive	Mediterranean-type Caucasian
V	Rarely burns, tans well, sun insensitive	Hispanic or Middle Eastern, possibly African-American
VI	Never burns, deeply pigmented, sun insensitive	African-American

you should consider wearing protective clothing and even lightweight gloves to shield the backs of your hands when you know that you're going to be outdoors for a prolonged period of time.

Even the daily commute requires some sun smarts, as UVA light can pass through car windows. Just 15 minutes of UVA exposure twice a day contributes to cumulative skin damage. We recommend installing a UVA shield on your windshield and the side windows, especially on the driver's side. You'll minimize not only skin damage but wrinkles and skin aging as well.

If you are taking any prescription or nonprescription medication, ask your physician or pharmacist if it can increase your sensitivity to the sun. Drugs such as tetracycline, ibuprofen, and certain antidepressants— along with herbs such as St. John's wort—can raise the risk of sunburn, regardless of skin type.

S U N S C R E E N
B Y   T H E   N U M B E R S

Two types of ultraviolet light play roles in skin cancer as well as in pho-
toaging—that is, skin changes such as fine wrinkles and brown spots that
result from sun exposure. Of the two, UVA has the longer wavelength,
and so can penetrate deep into the skin. For years UVA was thought to
be harmless, since so much of it is necessary to cause sunburn. Now it has
been implicated in melanoma, the deadliest form of skin cancer. It affects
the immune system, too.

Sun Protection for the Younger Set

Estimates are that between 50 and 80 percent of lifetime sun exposure occurs
by age 16. That's more than enough to set the stage for skin cancer, including melanoma.

Since scientists now believe that a bad sunburn early in life raises the risk
of skin cancer later on, you should take all precautions to safeguard the skin
of the children in your family. Keeping a youngster swabbed in sunscreen
won't do the job.

According to a survey of more than 500 Chicago households, most parents
had been using sunscreen on their children, yet 13 percent of the kids got
sunburns anyway. One explanation is that the parents had relied on sunscreen alone for protection, despite the fact that their children were
spending much more time in the sun than children who were not wearing
sunscreen. Using sunscreen may have created a false sense of security. Perhaps the parents had not made enough of an effort to keep their children in
the shade or to make them wear hats and protective clothing.

In fact, sunscreen is not the first-choice preventive measure for babies less
than 6 months old. But the American Academy of Pediatrics has issued a
statement saying that when adequate clothing—meaning long pants and a
long-sleeved shirt—and shade are not available, parents can apply a minimal

Because UVB has a shorter wavelength than UVA, it doesn't penetrate as deeply into the skin. Nevertheless, it is responsible for painful burning of the top layers. Research has linked UVB to basal and squamous cell carcinomas. (Incidentally, UVC—which has the shortest wavelength—is absorbed in the atmosphere and so never reaches the skin.)

Understanding the types of ultraviolet light is important because you want to choose a sunscreen that provides protection from both UVA and UVB rays. Not all of them do.

The government requires that all sunscreens be labeled with their sun protection factor, or SPF. These numbers have become so much a

amount of sunscreen on small areas, like the face and the backs of the hands. The academy also reminds parents that all children, including infants, should wear hats and sunglasses designed to block at least 99 percent of the sun's harmful ultraviolet rays.

Protecting older children can be more of a challenge. In persuading them to wear sunscreen and a hat and to stay in the shade as much as possible, stressing what is necessary to avoid the pain of sunburn likely will be much more effective than cautioning about the risk of skin cancer. Be sure your kids have hats that they will want to wear, and put sunscreen in their backpacks or beach bags before they head out.

The American Academy of Dermatology uses the abbreviation ABCS to teach children about sun protection.

- **A for *away***—stay away from the sun in the middle of the day.
- **B for *block***—use sunscreen with an SPF of 15 or higher, and reapply after swimming and/or every 2 hours, possibly more when sweating heavily.
- **C for *cover up***—wear a light-colored T-shirt and a hat.
- **S for *speak out***—talk to family and friends about sun protection.

part of our awareness that we toss them around with abandon—15 for day-to-day use, 30 for the beach. What many people don't realize is that the number is relevant only to UVB rays. Remember, most sunburn results from exposure to UVB, not UVA.

SPF is a measure of approximately how much time you can spend in the sun before burning. For example, if your skin is likely to burn in just 10 minutes when you're not wearing sunscreen, wearing an SPF 15 sunscreen will extend the time to burn to about 150 minutes (10 minutes × 15 = 150 minutes). For best protection, you should reapply the sunscreen every 2 hours (120 minutes).

A common assumption is that a higher SPF offers proportionately greater protection from the sun, but this isn't necessarily true. The differences in protection time tend to decrease as SPF increases. So wearing an SPF 50 sunscreen doesn't mean that you can stay out in the sun all day without burning.

Most health authorities recommend using a sunscreen with an SPF of at least 15 on a daily basis. An SPF 15 product provides adequate protection for most people who don't burn easily or on cloudy days. But if you're going to be in bright sunlight or you burn easily, we recommend going a little higher, to SPF 30. An SPF 30 product absorbs about 97 percent of the sun's UVB rays, compared with about 93 percent for SPF 15. What's more, SPF 30 protects against some, though not all, UVA rays. Besides, using a higher SPF offers extra insurance against applying too little sunscreen. (We'll say more in just a bit about how much sunscreen is enough.)

The shortcoming of an SPF 30 sunscreen is that it doesn't protect against all harmful UVA rays *unless* it contains an ingredient that specifically absorbs or blocks UVA. Since there are no established standards for labeling sunscreens or assessing a product's ability to shield against UVA rays, you need to know what to look for. Most sunscreen manufacturers use the phrase "broad-spectrum" on their labels to denote products with a UVA-protecting ingredient. Some use "UVA radiation protection," which means the same thing.

Studies have shown that UVA-protecting ingredients vary in their effectiveness. In general, products that contain zinc oxide or titanium dioxide, which block both UVA and UVB rays, or avobenzone (Parsol 1789), which absorbs UVA, work best. Another ingredient, Mexoryl, is available in Europe and is expected to soon be approved in the United States.

People who are sensitive or allergic to some of the chemical ingredients in sunscreens may not have the same adverse reactions to products made with micronized zinc oxide or titanium dioxide. Because the particles are so small, the products don't look white on the skin, yet they effectively block UVA and UVB rays.

HOW TO
APPLY SUNSCREEN

No sunscreen will safeguard against the sun's burning UVB rays or the deeply damaging UVA rays if you don't use it properly. This means applying a lot, applying early, and applying often. If you spend a cumulative 20 minutes outdoors on an average day, you need to wear sunscreen on all exposed areas—usually your face, ears, neck, and arms, and possibly your scalp—every day, even cloudy ones.

The laboratory tests that establish the SPF for sunscreen products use a larger amount of lotion, gel, or cream than is typical in real life. To get the amount of protection that you see on the label, you must apply sunscreen generously—something that 25 to 75 percent of people neglect to do, according to studies.

If you're heading to the pool or the beach, for instance, you should slather about a palmful or a shot-glass-ful of lotion on the exposed areas of your body 15 to 30 minutes before you leave home. Reapply the sunscreen 20 minutes after you're outside, and again after swimming and/or every 2 hours—more often if you perspire heavily. Be sure to rub the lotion in several different directions so you cover every square inch of exposed skin. Even waterproof sunscreens, which are formulated to maintain their SPF for 80 minutes in the water, need to be reapplied if you're swimming for any length of time. (Water-resistant sunscreens maintain their SPF for 40 minutes in the water.)

Be sure to protect your lips, too. Sunscreen-containing lip balms are widely available these days. Choose one with an SPF of 30 or higher.

If you haven't been shopping for sunscreen lately, you may be surprised by the sheer number of products on the market, in every form and price range. Some people buy different products for different occasions—perhaps one for wearing under makeup, one to use on the beach, and yet another for when playing sports. Whatever makes using sunscreen easy for you is what we recommend.

Keep in mind that while sunscreen will reduce your risk of skin cancer, no single product can provide complete 100 percent protection for your skin. This is why you also should follow our earlier recommendations to wear protective clothing *and* stay in the shade as much as you can.

THE HEALTHY TAN MYTH

Sun exposure triggers the production of melanin, the natural protective pigment in the skin. The increase in melanin is what creates a tan. It's true that a tan provides a kind of natural shield against the sun's ultraviolet rays. It's also true that tanning is a natural response to injury. In other words, once you have the tan, you've damaged your skin.

Sometimes tanning salons promote safe tanning without burning because tanning beds rely on UVA rays. But as we mentioned earlier, UVA rays still damage DNA and suppress your natural immunity. In one study, which involved nearly 1,000 people with basal cell or squamous cell carcinomas, those who had used a sun lamp or a tanning bed were 2½ times more likely to develop squamous cell carcinomas and 1½ times more likely to develop basal cell carcinomas than those who hadn't used an artificial tanning device. Interestingly, people who had been advised to avoid the sun—perhaps because they burned easily—were more likely to try sun lamps and tanning beds, thinking they could tan safely.

Cosmetic scientists may have come up with the perfect solution for men and women who worship the sun: the sunless tanning product, which stains the skin in a way that looks like a natural tan. At last they can achieve a sun-burnished glow without risking skin cancer. Sunless tanning products for the face and body come in lotions, sprays, and gels. They've been perfected in recent years, so the streaking and spotting that once was a problem can be avoided with careful application. If you try one of these products, keep in mind that your man-made tan will not protect your skin from the sun's ultraviolet rays.

If your primary concern is not tanning but avoiding skin cancer, the American Cancer Society sums up the basics of sun protection in this easy-to-remember guideline: Slip on a shirt, slop on sunscreen, and slap on a hat.

SCHEDULE

YOUR

CANCER

CHECKUPS

* * * * * * * * *

ONE THING WE KNOW FOR CERTAIN about cancer: In most cases, the sooner it's detected, the more likely it can be cured. With regular checkups and the screening techniques currently available, some conditions that might lead to cancer can be caught early, and early-stage cancers can be treated before they advance.

Unfortunately, most people don't get checkups and screenings as often as they should, if at all. For example, in more than half of all cases of colorectal cancer, the disease already has spread in the region or to distant sites by the time it's diagnosed. Yet it could have been prevented entirely if the precancer—an intestinal polyp—had been detected and removed.

Similarly, the mammogram can identify cancerous changes in their earliest stages, before they turn into to full-blown breast cancer. But 30 percent of women over age 40 do not get mammograms every year, or even every 2 years.

We're fortunate to live in an era when an amazing array of tools and techniques can catch cancer early on. But these screening tests will save lives only if people get them at specific recommended intervals. Institutions, agencies, and organizations may vary in their screening guidelines, but they share one objective: early detection.

SCREENING IS NOT DIAGNOSIS

It's important to understand that in general, screening tests—which detect abnormal cells or growths—are different from diagnostic tests. If a screening test finds anything suspicious, a diagnostic test often follows.

A positive result on a screening test, or the appearance of an abnormality, doesn't necessarily mean that you have cancer. It does mean that you need further evaluation, with more testing. Usually it involves the removal of abnormal cells for a biopsy. The cells are examined under a microscope to determine whether any are cancerous.

In some tests, such as colonoscopy, doctors can retrieve a sample of tissue from an abnormal area during the screening procedure for follow-up examination. Other tests, such as mammography, require a separate biopsy to diagnose or rule out a malignancy.

Since diagnostic tests are beyond the scope of this book, we have not included extensive descriptions of the signs and symptoms of cancer. In general, we recommend seeing your physician if you notice anything unusual, such as blood in the stool, vaginal bleeding after menopause, any abnormal bleeding or discharge, a lump or growth anywhere on the body, or unexplained fatigue or weight loss.

WHICH TESTS DO YOU NEED?

The recommended frequency of your screening tests will depend largely on your individual risk, which is why you and your doctor need to evaluate your risk factors for all the major cancers. If you're of average risk, then the screening guidelines presented in chapter 4 likely will be sufficient. If you're of above-average risk—based on your family history, your personal history, and/or your lifestyle choices—you and your doctor should decide which screening tests you need and how often.

Sometimes physicians recommend additional screening tests for patients who are at high risk for certain kinds of cancer. Some of these tests—such as the blood test for CA-125, a marker for ovarian cancer—have a high rate of false-positive results, so they are not useful for the general population. But they might be appropriate for you.

Another possibility is to enroll in a clinical trial of a screening test, like the one currently under way to assess the usefulness of CT scans in detecting lung cancer in smokers. Other clinical trials are studying variations on or combinations of screening tests already in wide use. (To learn more about these trials, refer to the individual cancer chapters in part 2.)

The American Cancer Society recommends a cancer-related checkup every 3 years for men and women between ages 20 and 39, and every year for those ages 40 and older. During this checkup, your physician will conduct an examination for signs of cancer of the skin, lymph nodes, oral cavity, ovaries, breast, and colon, among other things. He may perform certain screening tests during this exam. And he probably will ask questions about your health habits and lifestyle, to identify potential cancer risk factors. This is an excellent opportunity for you to ask questions about your individual cancer risk, and to find out whether you're a candidate for other screening tests that are not considered routine.

Once you schedule an appointment for your cancer-related checkup, plan ahead. Considering how medical practices have changed, especially in terms of the limited "face time" between patient and physician, try to be as organized as you can. Make a list of your questions. If you have a particular concern that may require lengthier discussion—whether to undergo certain genetic testing, for example—make an appointment for that purpose specifically.

While we're on the subject of cancer-related checkups, we want to stress the importance of having a primary care physician and, for women, a gynecologist. Studies show that women who receive regular medical care are more likely to have mammograms and Pap tests. The same may hold true for men, who can get rectal exams from their primary care physicians, ideally as part of their regular cancer-related checkups. If they happen to develop urinary symptoms, they may receive a referral to a urologist for further evaluation.

WHAT TO DO BEFORE AND AFTER

Keep a schedule of screening tests in your daily planner or electronic calendar, as a reminder to make the necessary appointments well in advance. Because the tests occur at varying intervals, you should establish some sort of system to track which test you need and when. For example, some women plan their mammograms around their birth dates because it's easy to remember (though if you are perimenopausal, try to make your mammogram appointment for after your period). Tests that are less frequent, such as sigmoidoscopy, may be more easily forgotten.

Studies have found that physicians vary in their knowledge of cancer screening guidelines, so we suggest doing some homework of your own. The American Cancer Society, for example, has established screening guidelines for the major types of cancer. While we refer to these guidelines throughout this book, you may want to call (800) ACS-2345 or visit the ACS Web site (www.cancer.org) to stay up-to-date on changes.

You also may want to find out which screening tests your health plan covers. Fortunately, insurers have become much more accommodating in this regard. Still, the co-payments can add up, and you'll need to be financially prepared. But don't let the out-of-pocket costs discourage you from getting the necessary screenings. Give your body the same respectful treatment that you give your car or your home. You wouldn't forgo changing your oil or fixing a leaky roof because you didn't want to spend the money. So why forgo your screening tests?

Prior to testing, do what you can to ensure the accuracy of the results. This means following any preparation instructions to the letter. If in doubt, call beforehand for clarification on any aspect of the preparation process that you don't understand. Yes, the prework may be inconvenient or time-consuming. But to avoid repeating a test, you need to get it right the first time.

Just as important as following through on the screening tests is following up afterward. Most likely, you will need to call your doctor and request your test results. Otherwise, any number of events—from misplaced reports to unforwarded phone messsages—could prevent the information from reaching you. Some physicians and medical centers routinely mail test results so their patients have a written record for their personal medical files. If your doctor doesn't do this, you may want to ask if he could.

If you're asked to repeat a screening test or to have another type of test as a follow-up, do it. Chances are your doctor noticed some irregu-

Your Screening Test Schedule

Many cancer experts espouse the American Cancer Society guidelines for screening tests. We've summarized these guidelines here, by age. You may want to make a copy of this chart to keep with your personal medical records or your daily planner. When you see your doctor for your cancer checkup, review the chart and modify it according to your unique risk profile.

AGE	SCREENING TEST	FREQUENCY
3 years after becoming sexually active, but no later than age 21	Pap test	Every year for conventional tests; every 2 years for liquid-based tests
20–39	Cancer-related checkup	Every 3 years
	Clinical breast exam	Every 3 years
	Breast self-exam	Monthly, if desired
	Pap test	Same as above, except after age 30; then if three consecutive Pap tests produce normal results, the interval between tests may extend to every 2–3 years
		For women over age 30, an alternative to the Pap test alone is the Pap test in combination an HPV DNA test; if both tests come back negative, the interval between screenings may extend to every 3 years

larity that needs confirmation or further evaluation. Follow-up is part of the screening process and should never be ignored. Remember that most abnormalities turn out to not be cancer.

TAKE CARE NOT TO OVERDO

Some people believe that they need certain screening tests more often than most guidelines suggest. If you are considering extra testing, discuss

AGE	SCREENING TEST	FREQUENCY
40–49	Skin self-exam	Periodically
	Cancer-related checkup	Every year
	Clinical breast exam	Every year
	Mammography	Every year
	Breast self-exam	Monthly, if desired
	Pap test	Same as above
50 and older	*In addition to the above tests:* PSA test and digital rectal exam	Discuss with your doctor whether you should have a PSA test and, if so, how often
	Colon and rectal cancer screening	One of the following: fecal occult blood test (FOBT) every year; flexible sigmoidoscopy every 5 years; FOBT every year plus flexible sigmoidoscopy every 5 years (both are preferable to either one alone); double-contrast barium enema every 5 years; colonoscopy every 10 years
70 and older	Pap test	May be discontinued after three consecutive tests with normal results and no abnormal results in 10 years

the matter with your doctor. Depending on your risk, more frequent screenings may be a good idea. But unnecessary screening tests raise the chances of a false-positive result, which in turn may lead to unnecessary diagnostic testing.

These days, freestanding screening centers are opening in malls and shopping centers across the country, and they're marketing CT and MRI scans—primarily to detect cancer and heart disease—directly to consumers. Although these imaging tests can identify abnormal growths in the body, they seldom can distinguish between a benign lesion and a malignant one. Therefore, widespread use of this technology could lead to a significant number of false-positive results and unnecessary surgical biopsies.

Some experts believe these imaging tests also create a false sense of security among people who have them. Someone who gets an all-clear as a result of a CT scan at the mall may decide to skip the routine screening tests that could be more effective in detecting some types of cancer. Furthermore, the imaging tests carry risks of their own. For instance, a CT scan emits 70 times as much radiation dose as a single chest x-ray.

A study is under way to determine whether a new type of imaging, called a spiral CT scan, is a cost-effective means of detecting lung cancer in smokers. Until the study is complete, and until others determine the best way to use this imaging tool, we don't recommend spiral CT scan for healthy people as a means of detecting lung cancer.

So which screening tests provide the best chance of identifying pre-cancers and early-stage cancers? And how often should you have them? We suggest following the American Cancer Society guidelines, which we've summarized in the chart on page 272. These guidelines establish a basic screening program for early detection; you and your doctor may customize it to fit your unique risk profile.

FIGHTING FEAR

Perhaps one of the significant obstacles to routine cancer screenings is fear—of the disease, of the treatment, of the prognosis. Sometimes it seems that people would rather not know that they have cancer, perhaps not realizing that they could be missing out on an opportunity to arrest the disease in its earliest stages. Research has shown that personal and cultural beliefs about cancer can have a profound impact on whether a person is willing to do what's necessary for early detection of the disease.

If you find yourself putting off a mammogram or a colonoscopy, for example, think about why you're doing it. Explore the source of your fear and learn more about the object of your concern. Yet while knowledge can go a long way in dispelling fear, you may need to just muster your courage and take action. Perhaps asking a trusted family member or friend to join you will take some of the sting out of the process.

THE BEST

MEDICINE

• • • • • • • • •

Throughout this book, we've outlined strategies that can help protect virtually anyone against all kinds of cancer. For those at especially high risk for certain cancers, we've identified measures to address their special needs. All of this information draws on what we know now about cancer prevention. Future advances will provide further proof that prevention is the best cancer fighter around. And they'll show with greater precision just how much you can lower your risk.

For instance, you now know that obesity is a risk factor for a number of cancers. But ongoing research may reveal just how many pounds a person who's overweight would need to lose to improve his or her risk profile. We already know that just a 10 percent reduction in body weight can lower the risk of diabetes; will the same hold true for cancer? Likewise, several nutrition trials currently underway will help determine which fruits and vegetables are most important for cancer prevention, particularly for specific cancers. And of course, developments in the field of chemoprevention promise to revolutionize how doctors help people at very high risk for the disease.

While many exciting breakthroughs lie ahead, you don't need to wait for them to take action. We hope that you will use the information in this book to make smart choices that will help you stay healthy and cancer-free for life.

INDEX

C • • •

CA-125, indicating ovarian cancer, 34, 170–71, 172–73

CA19-9, indicating pancreatic cancer, 184

Calcium, for cancer prevention, 63–64, 161, 175

Calorie cutting, for weight loss, 229–31

Cancer-related checkups, 36, 270–71

Cancer survivors, preventing recurrence in, 29–30

Capsule video endoscopy, for detecting colorectal cancer, 160–61

Carcinogens
definition of, 9
in grilled meat, 46
job-related, 52, 53
Web site on, 53

Caucasians, cancer in. *See* Whites, cancer in

Celebrex. *See* Celecoxib

Celecoxib
for preventing
breast cancer, 133–34
colorectal cancer, 56, 162–63, 212
lung cancer, 146
oral cancer, 206–7
skin cancer, 91
for treating colon polyps, xi, 61–62

Cell division, in cancer, 3–4

Cells
in cancer formation, 5–6
categories of, for cancer identification, 6

Cellular analysis, for cancer prevention, 33–34

Cervical cancer
in African-Americans, 187
in Asian-Americans, 29
causes of, 2, 39, 49, 50, 190–91, 212
chemoprevention for, 196–97
death rate from, 187

decline in, 187
in Hispanics, 28
incidence of, 187
preventing, xiii, 72, 195–96, 198
risk factors for, 188–90, 191, 255
screening guidelines for, 36–37, 38–39
screening tests for
colposcopy, 194–95
HPV DNA testing, 194
Pap test, 7, 35, 36–37, 39, 55–56, 187, 190, 191–94

Cervix, anatomy and function of, **189**

Characteristics of cancer, 5–6

Chemoprevention, x–xi, 6, 75–77. *See also* Chemopreventives
for breast cancer, 65–72, 76, 132–35
for cervical cancer, 196–97
for colorectal cancer, 162–63
future of, 73
for lung cancer, 146
for melanoma, 90–92
for oral cancer, 33, 205–7
for ovarian cancer, 177–78
overview of, 54–57
for pancreatic cancer, 185
for prostate cancer, 102–4

Chemopreventives. *See also* Chemoprevention
classes of, 57
calcium, 63–64
cyclooxygenase inhibitors, 60–63
hormone blockers, 64–72
retinoids, 58–60
vaccines, 72

Chest x-rays, for detecting lung cancer, 143–44

Childbearing, late, as breast cancer risk factor, 108

Chlamydia, as cervical cancer risk factor, 188, 191, 255